CRITICAL THINKING IN PRACTICAL/ VOCATIONAL NURSING

Lois White, RN, PhD

Former Chairperson, Professor
Department of Vocational Nurse Education
Del Mar College
Corpus Christi, Texas

DELMAR

™

THOMSON LEARNING

Australia Canada Mexico Singapore Spain United Kingdom United States

Delmar Staff:
Business Unit Director: William Brottmiller
Executive Editor: Cathy L. Esperti
Acquisitions Editor: Matthew Filimonov
Editorial Assistant: Melissa Longo
Executive Marketing Manager: Dawn F. Gerrain
Channel Manager: Tara Carter
Art/Design Coordinator: Tim Conners

Printed in the United States
1 2 3 4 5 XXX 05 04 03 02 01

For more information, contact Delmar,
3 Columbia Circle, PO Box 15015, Albany, NY 12212-0515

Or find us on the World Wide Web at http://www.delmar.com

Library of Congress Cataloging-in-Publication Data
White, Lois.
      Critical thinking in practical/vocational nursing / Lois White.
         p. cm.
      Includes index.
      ISBN 0-7668-3458-1 (alk. paper)
         1. Nursing—Study and teaching—Problems, exercises, etc.
2. Critical thinking Problems, exercises, etc. I. Title.

RT73 .W48 2001
610.73'076—dc21   2001028770

Notice to the Reader

Contents

Chapter 1 Critical Thinking 1
Critical Thinking 2
Skills of Critical Thinking 6
Standards for Critical Thinking 11
Reasoning and Problem-Solving 16
Traits of a Disciplined Thinker 21
Critical Thinking in Nursing 23

Chapter 2 Skills for Success 35
Develop a Positive Attitude 37
Develop Your Basic Skills 43
Develop Your Learning Style 52
Develop a Time-Management Plan 57
Develop a Study Strategy 64
Practice Thinking Critically 76
Develop Test-Taking Skills 78

Appendix A: Nursing Practice Standards for the
   Licensed Practical/Vocational Nurse 99
Appendix B: Answer Key 105
Glossary 107
Index 109

Preface

The ability to think on one's feet is crucial for today's nurses. Roles and responsibilities are continually shifting as the health care environment evolves. Clients need change as well.

Everyone acknowledges that critical thinking is important. Unfortunately, there is often a great deal of confusion as to exactly what critical thinking is or how to integrate it into the classroom. This situation is further complicated by the tremendous amount of information that instructors are expected to teach students.

Critical Thinking in Practical/Vocational Nursing was developed to help instructors include a discussion of critical thinking and study skills concepts in their classrooms. A review of these important concepts at the beginning of any student's nursing education will help the student succeed and excel.

Organization

The book is divided into two convenient sections:

Chapter 1: Critical Thinking. This chapter lays the groundwork for learning. It outlines the process of critical thinking in easy-to-understand terms, offering students tips and exercises for comprehension. By teaching students "how to think" about nursing and how to solve nursing problems, students will be better prepared to succeed in their studies.

"I, for lack of a better word, 'loved' the chapters. After reading them I began to understand why our students 'just don't get it' sometimes. We give them the critical thinking exercises and assignments to do. But who has taught them how to think critically? I love the example of trying to play soccer without knowing the rules of the game; it really hit home hard. We are asking our students to do something that they haven't been taught to do."

Kathy White, RN

Chapter 2: Skills for Success. This final chapter focuses on strategies for learning and studying that may not be readily apparent to struggling students.

"This concept is one that is being encouraged by my peers as critical to success in nursing. There are many students who lack these life skills when they enter nursing."

Kay Rice Francis, RN, MSN

About the Author

Lois Elain Wacker White earned a diploma in nursing from Memorial Hospital School of Nursing, Springfield, Illinois; an Associate degree in Science from Del Mar College, Corpus Christi, Texas; a Bachelor of Science in Nursing from Texas A & I University-Corpus Christi, Corpus Christi, Texas; a Master of Science in Education from Corpus Christi State University, Corpus Christi, Texas; and a Doctor of Philosophy degree in educational administration-community college from the University of Texas, Austin, Texas.

She has taught at Del Mar College, Corpus Christi, Texas, in both the Associate Degree Nursing program and the Vocational Nursing program. For 14 years she was also chairperson of the Department of Vocational Nurse Education. Dr. White has taught fundamentals of nursing, nutrition, mental health/mental illness, medical–surgical nursing, and maternal/newborn nursing. Her professional career has also included 15 years of clinical practice.

Dr. White has served on the Nursing Education Advisory Committee of the Board of Nurse Examiners for the State of Texas and the Board of Vocational Nurse Examiners, which developed competencies expected of graduates from each level of nursing. She maintains membership in the Texas Association of Vocational Nurse Educators, Sigma Theta Tau, American Nurses Association, and the National League for Nursing.

Dr. White has been listed in *Who's Who in American Nursing*. She currently serves on the Vocational Nursing Financial Aid Advisory Committee for the Texas Higher Education Coordinating Board.

Reviewers

Kay Rice Francis
Lake Michigan College

Kathy White
Missouri Delta Medical Center

Patty Leary
Mecosta Osceola ISD — Career Center

Carol Nelson
Spokane Community College

CRITICAL THINKING

Upon completion of this chapter, you should be able to:
- *Define key terms.*
- *State five characteristics of the person who uses critical thinking.*
- *Identify behaviors that illustrate the traits of a nurse who is a critical thinker.*
- *Assess personal strengths and weaknesses in relation to critical thinking skills.*
- *Develop a personal plan for the enhancement of personal critical thinking and reasoning skills.*

KEY TERMS

concept	judgment	reasoning
critical thinking	justify	reflective
discipline	logic	standard
disciplined	opinion	

INTRODUCTION

Thinking as a nurse involves much more than gathering an assortment of facts and skills. Critical thinking in nursing education is not a separate component of the curriculum. It is "an approach to inquiry where both students and faculty examine clinical and professional issues and search for more effective answers" (Miller & Malcolm, 1990).

Nursing is part of a rapidly changing and increasingly complex society. Anyone who expects to have a successful career in nursing, at any level, must be able to compete effectively. This means that practical/vocational nurses must have good problem-solving skills and make quality decisions related to the client care they deliver. Over the past 15 years, increasing attention has been paid to the need for graduates of educational programs at every level and in every **discipline** (branch of learning, field of study, or occupation requiring specialized knowledge) to develop better thinking skills. Nurse educators have been among the leaders in the current movement to find ways to improve the thinking ability of their students. Nurses in clinical practice have also been challenged to improve their ability to reason clearly and logically. Because of these movements, you, as a beginning nursing student, will need to develop your critical thinking skills.

CRITICAL THINKING

The first step in improving your ability to think well is to develop an understanding of **critical thinking**. This involves much more than memorizing a simple definition of this process. The ability to think critically requires a great deal of effort and time. There are many definitions, all of which may be valuable, as you begin the process of learning to assess your own thinking and the quality of the thinking of others (see Figure 1-1). In fact, memorizing an exact definition of critical thinking would be detrimental to the full development of an understanding of this **disciplined** (trained by instruction and exercise) type of thinking. The **concept** of critical thinking includes the basic idea that one becomes a better thinker by developing specific attitudes, traits, and skills. A concept is a mental picture of abstract phenomena that serves to organize observations related to that phenomena. Each person must learn to be **reflective**, or introspective, about his or her own thinking. Critical thinking was briefly described in this way in a workshop presented by Richard Paul (Paul & Willsen, 1993): "Critical thinking is that mode of thinking—about any subject, content, or problem—in which the thinker improves the quality of his or her thinking by skillfully taking charge of the structures inherent in thinking and imposing intellectual **standards** (or a level or degree of quality) upon them." To ensure integrity and consistency of the presentation in this chapter, the criteria, standards, and materials

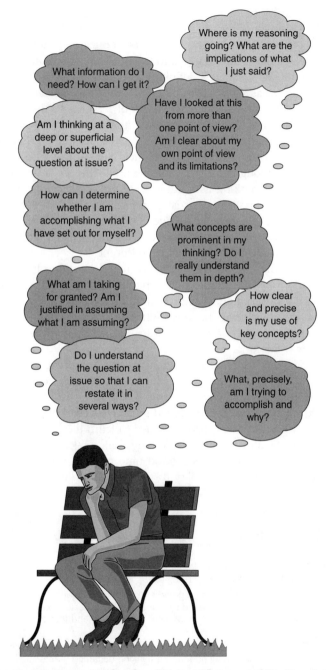

Figure 1-1 Assessing Our Own Thinking (*Courtesy of The Foundation for Critical Thinking, Dillon Beach, CA*)

developed by the Center for Critical Thinking have been used as the organizing framework.

In a newsletter designed for nurse educators interested in the use of critical thinking within the nursing curriculum, Penny Heaslip (1994) presents a definition of critical thinking. This definition serves as a basis for you to develop strategies and tactics as you begin the exciting experience of learning to think more clearly, and in a disciplined manner, about nursing. A comprehensive definition of critical thinking is the disciplined, intellectual process of applying skillful clinical **reasoning** (use of the elements of thought to solve a problem or settle a question) and self-reflective thinking as a guide to belief or action in nursing practice (Heaslip, 1994; Norris & Ennis, 1989; Paul, 1990).

Table 1-1 presents some definitions of critical thinking. Review them and compare the elements that are common to all of them and the elements that are different.

Most of the authors who have written about critical thinking have addressed instructors. This chapter is written for you, the student. It is designed to guide your process of reflecting on and evaluating your own thinking. While your instructors want to help you with the process, you are ultimately responsible for your own thinking.

Many students enter nursing programs unprepared to think critically. Many educators believe this inability may be the result of a lack of instruction in thinking. The result is similar to what would happen to you if you tried to play soccer without knowing the rules or having had a chance to learn the basic skills of the game. Quality thinking is like any skill; it takes practice and discipline to learn. This is a good time to do a self-evaluation related to your current ability to perform the four basic critical

Table 1-1 DEFINITIONS OF CRITICAL THINKING

- "Reflective and reasonable thinking that is focused on deciding what to believe or do" (Ennis, 1985).
- "An investigation whose purpose is to explore a situation, phenomenon, question, or problem to arrive at a hypothesis or conclusion about it that integrates all available information and that can therefore be convincingly justified" (Kurfiss, 1988).
- "The attentive commitment to a self-reflective process of examining one's thoughts, ensuring that the thinking occurring meets intellectual standards" (Heaslip, 1993).

thinking processes: reading for meaning, listening critically, writing clearly, and speaking in a logical, coherent manner. These four skills are discussed in the next section. If your basic education program did not emphasize all of these skills, decide now to develop these abilities.

New Information

The quantity of new information that you must be prepared to master may be a barrier to the development of critical thinking skills. Many students (and instructors) focus so intently on the content of a course that they allow little time to think about the material. The ability to think critically about the knowledge base of nursing is essential for learning the content of your nursing courses. The discipline of nursing has an organizing **logic**, or formal principles of a branch of knowledge, that serves to define the appropriate facts and methods required to produce effective nursing practice. This logic serves as a framework within which the student can construct a unique, meaningful system for the practice of nursing. Your nursing program probably has a philosophy and a statement of the main concepts that the nursing faculty use to present the course material in a logical framework.

Activity

If you have not yet reviewed your program's philosophy and main concepts for the purpose of helping you understand your program of study, this would be a good time to do so. Most programs of nursing include a philosophy statement, organizing concepts, and program outcomes in the student handbook or other document provided to students. These resources can help you use your own logic to discover the logic of nursing as presented in your program. Try the following activities:

1. Identify the major concepts (such as nursing, learning, caring) that provide structure for your program's philosophy and organization.
2. Discuss the components, or parts, of each major theme with your classmates and instructors.
3. Use your own words to see how your mental pictures of these ideas may be the same or different from those in your program materials.
4. Review the material you have already covered in your nursing program to identify how the major parts of each course relate to these concepts.

5. Look at the objectives for this course and the topics in this textbook to see how they will relate to the main ideas you have discovered in this activity.

Student Responsibility

Finally, many students find the process of becoming responsible for their own thinking painful. For many students the education processes that were part of their basic school preparation were based on a very structured approach to acquiring selected facts and skills; the students' recall was then tested by "objective" tests. If this was your experience, you may view learning as being the result of the teacher's presenting what must be learned and devising "fair" tests. You may thus believe that your own input to the learning process is less important than that of the teacher. You, along with many other students, may find that you are uncomfortable when asked to decide what is important or to be able to defend your **opinions** (subjective beliefs) and **judgments** (conclusions based on sound reasoning and supported by evidence). You may prefer to be told, with no ambiguity, what you need to know.

Nursing, however, does not take place in predictable, highly structured situations. Practical/vocational nurses are required to make decisions at many levels. Knowing how to make good decisions begins with developing the essential skills, traits, and attitudes associated with critical thinking.

SKILLS OF CRITICAL THINKING

Four basic skills are necessary for the development of higher-level thinking skills. These skills are part of the process of developing and using thinking for problem-solving and reasoning. Your abilities in these four areas can be measured by the extent to which you are achieving the universal intellectual standards (UIS). These standards are discussed in the following section and are illustrated in Table 1-2. The four basic skills are critical reading, critical listening, critical writing, and critical speaking.

Critical Reading

Reading for meaning is basic to the acquisition of knowledge from textbooks and journals. The student who can read critically

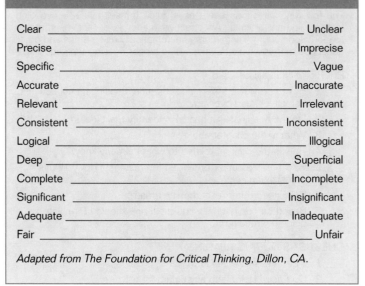

Table 1-2 **THE SPECTRUM OF UNIVERSAL INTELLECTUAL STANDARDS**

Clear	Unclear
Precise	Imprecise
Specific	Vague
Accurate	Inaccurate
Relevant	Irrelevant
Consistent	Inconsistent
Logical	Illogical
Deep	Superficial
Complete	Incomplete
Significant	Insignificant
Adequate	Inadequate
Fair	Unfair

Adapted from The Foundation for Critical Thinking, Dillon, CA.

will also do better on tests. Study time will be reduced and retention of material will be enhanced. An exercise that can help build reading skills is to use a highlighter pen to mark the main idea of a sentence. Students who have not learned to read critically will find that they have marked most of the text. Joining a study group may help you identify main ideas by comparing with others the various main ideas each of you have derived from the same material. During test reviews, you can make sure to note when misreading or misinterpretation caused you to make an error on the test. By making a conscious effort to identify your individual weaknesses, you will improve your critical reading skills.

Another tactic you can try is to practice restating the main idea to yourself or to another student. As you read the text, have a dialogue with yourself, which could go something like this: "What is the reason for studying this material? How does this relate to what I already know? This does not seem to fit. Did I misunderstand? Can I say this in my own words?" Worrell (1990) has developed a useful tool for guiding your dialogue. It is illustrated in Table 1-3.

Table 1-3 STRATEGIC READING LIST

The following questions serve as a guide for self-talk when reading texts or journal articles. An effective reader is an active, strategic reader! Soon you will find yourself automatically using these and other questions that you have developed, no longer needing the checklist.

PREREADING QUESTIONS

___ 1. Have I previewed (skimmed) the title, headings, subheadings, objectives, and overview?

___ 2. Do the headings/subheadings identify main ideas?

___ 3. What is the chapter about?

___ 4. How is the content related to what I already know?

___ 5. How has the author organized the material? How will this organization help me?

___ 6. Will I need other resources as I read?

___ 7. Based on previewing, what questions should I formulate to guide my reading?

QUESTIONS DURING READING

___ 1. Does this make sense to me?

___ 2. Do I need to look up any unfamiliar words?

___ 3. Do I need to reread difficult material? Or will this be explained further if I read on?

___ 4. Is the author using signal words (*first, next, therefore, as a result,* etc.)?

___ 5. How is this information related to what I know?

___ 6. How is this section linked to the previous section?

___ 7. Can I summarize this section before going any further?

___ 8. Can I answer my prereading questions? Can I formulate new questions?

QUESTIONS AFTER READING

___ 1. Do I understand the main points?

___ 2. Can I outline the content?

___ 3. How is this related to previous learning?

___ 4. How would I use or apply this information?

___ 5. Are there points that I need to clarify? How will I do this?

___ 6. What questions would likely be on an exam from this material?

___ 7. Can I answer my questions, paraphrase the content, and link main points without looking at my notes or text?

From Metacognition: Implications for Instruction in Nursing Education, *by P. J. Worrell, 1990,* Journal of Nursing Education, 29(4).
Reprinted with permission of Journal of Nursing Education, *SLACK Incorporated, Thorofare, NJ.*

Critical Listening

Communication skills, especially listening skills, receive a great deal of emphasis in the nursing curriculum. Even so, many persons do not have effective listening skills. One reason is that many persons have developed the habit of tuning in only occasionally to orally presented material. The result is that the meaning of the oral communication is lost. A way to improve your listening skills is to try to restate the points made in a discussion with another student and have that student give feedback about how accurately you have restated her position. Critical listening also requires that you carry on a mental dialogue with the speaker. For instance, as you listen, focus on what the speaker is saying, listen for key points, notice anything that seems confusing to you as well as those points you already understand (Figure 1-2).

Critical listening requires that you make a conscious commitment to focus on the topic of discussion. This means that you should actively attend to the words and meanings of the speaker. Your ability to recognize things that distract your attention is valuable in increasing your listening skills. Some typical distractions for students include attempting to take word-for-word notes, focusing on the mannerisms or appearance of the speaker, and daydreaming. As in all areas, a good thinker is not afraid to identify weaknesses and strengths in order to improve.

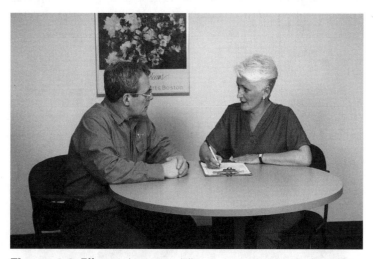

Figure 1-2 Effective listening skills are essential to all client interactions.

Critical Writing

The ability to state one's thoughts coherently, clearly, and concisely is basic to good thinking skills. Many students arrive at college unable to write well. The quality of thinking is improved by the discipline required to state facts and judgments well. Many students are afraid to write down their thoughts, because they feel that writing is too revealing. Writing is important for the improvement of thinking because it can be reviewed using the UIS to evaluate the quality of the thinking reflected in the writing (Figure 1-3). These standards are discussed in greater detail later in the chapter. You may also refer back to Table 1-2.

One technique for improving the quality of your thinking through writing is to summarize, in your own words, the main idea in a reading assignment. Next, use that main idea in relation to a client care problem from the material you are studying. Then, put the writing away until the next day and reread it. Can you understand it? Submit it to a friend for critique. Can your friend understand what you meant to say? How could you improve what you have written? Improving your writing skills may not seem like fun, but it is an effective and vital process for improving the quality of your own thinking.

Critical Speaking

Perhaps the most neglected skill is disciplined speaking. We do not hear many examples of clear, logical, accurate spoken communication. Oral communication is different from written

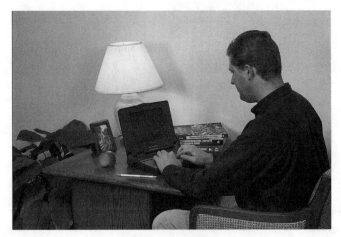

Figure 1-3 Effective writing skills are integral to critical thinking.

communication. It is usually more spontaneous and must be carefully presented because, unless recorded, it is present only for the moment. Ambiguous statements are misleading. Personal biases influence what the other person hears. Practicing in a small group and soliciting feedback from the listeners can help a student assess and improve this skill.

STANDARDS FOR CRITICAL THINKING

The simple definition of critical thinking used in the preceding section includes the provision that the assessment of your own thinking relies on the use of universal standards for quality thinking. As you begin to develop and apply critical thinking to nursing, the first requirement is to become familiar with these standards. The Spectrum of Universal Intellectual Standards developed by The Center for Critical Thinking is used in this discussion because it provides a valid and reliable measure for the quality of thinking. Whether you are reading the assigned material from a textbook, listening to an oral presentation, writing a paper, answering test questions, or presenting ideas in oral form, the following standards should be applied.

Clarity vs. Lack of Clarity

Fundamental to quality thinking is the ability to think clearly. Thinking clearly means that you can place the facts and ideas of course content into a logical and coherent framework. The measure for the degree to which this is true is the degree to which you can state these relationships orally or in writing so that others can understand your position. One tactic for increasing your clarity of thought is to pay particular attention to the exact meaning of the words encountered. The year that you spend in the practical/vocational nursing program is filled with many new terms and concepts. Time spent in practicing the proper use of these terms and in applying concepts appropriately will result in improved clarity of thought and increased retention of content. You can use small study groups to challenge one another to write and speak clearly as you review content together.

A review of the words used in the preceding paragraph may illustrate how the meaning of words can be misunderstood. For example, think about the word *clarity*. When you look up this word in a dictionary, you find that there are several shades of meaning. Look up the word for yourself and decide which of the definitions applies to the use of clarity in describing a standard for critical thinking.

Think about some expressions you use every day. Would someone who is from another part of the country understand them? An example is the use of the term *this evening,* which is common in some parts of the country. If someone told you that she would visit you "this evening," when would you expect her? In some places, the person might arrive in the early afternoon; in other places, at night. When speaking to clients, families, and other health team members, the nurse must be sure that the words used clearly express the intended message. When reading or listening, do not assume that you understand a term. Take the time to verify the meaning.

Precision vs. Imprecision

Sometimes, we have a "ballpark" mentality. That is, we learn enough about a subject to be "in the ballpark," but not enough to hit a home run. The result is a general idea of the meaning of a fact or idea, but not enough understanding to apply it or to use the information for problem-solving or promoting communication of an idea to someone else. You may be making this mistake if you find yourself saying something like this: "I knew that, but on the test, it was stated differently." Precision of thought means that the meaning of a concept is clearly understood in terms of its relationship to other concepts and to its practical implications, so that the thought is exact, accurate, and definite (Paul & Willsen, 1993).

Specificity vs. Vagueness

Specificity means that the student can be concrete or exact in stating or applying a fact. An example of vagueness, which can be commonly ascribed to nursing students, occurs during the use of the planning phase of the nursing process when students do not write concrete nursing interventions. For example, a student may state that the nursing action will "provide support to the client and his family." It is difficult to explain exactly what this statement means, either in general or in relation to this client and this nurse. Appropriate planning involves deciding on definite, well-stated nursing diagnoses, goals, and nursing actions. The use of the nursing process requires that the student learn the degree of specificity required for each nursing situation. State or itemize the nursing actions to be performed.

Accuracy vs. Inaccuracy

Accuracy means being correct and within the proper parameters. Nursing students can readily understand the need for accurate calculation of a drug dose or accurate measurement of blood pressure. In the same way, the collection and interpretation of data must be accurate. Accuracy usually implies the use of some measuring instrument. In the case of blood pressure, this is easy to see. In the case of accuracy in thinking, it may be harder to conceptualize. An example would be when the nurse uses the term *hypertension* to mean someone who is anxious and hyperactive instead of the actual meaning, an elevation of blood pressure above the accepted normal maximum. When dealing with more abstract concepts, accuracy of interpretation and understanding are equally important. Students can improve the accuracy of their thinking by trying to write new information in their own words and having another student interpret the meaning. Inaccurate information will become evident.

Accurate recording of findings during client care is essential to quality care. Accurate understanding of the concepts underlying each part of your nursing course, plus understanding how each part of your nursing course relates to any given client, will enable you to be more accurate in your thinking.

There are degrees of accuracy. For example, you might measure a client's temperature using a thermometer that can measure to the 0.01 degree, but this degree of accuracy may be unnecessary. On the other hand, when figuring a pediatric dosage, a difference of 0.01 can be important. One of your challenges is to increase your awareness of the degree of accuracy required in given nursing situations.

Relevance vs. Irrelevance

Relevance refers to needed information as opposed to information that is not needed at the moment. Students must be able to separate the two; otherwise, they may spend time arguing for a position that does not matter. For instance, students may get sidetracked from the purpose of an exercise by failing to limit their responses to the central issue or heart of the question or problem to be solved. It is also important to be able to recognize when sufficient relevant information is not available. An example of failing to recognize relevant information might be ignoring a client's comment that his rash began the day after starting a new medication. On the other hand, the nurse may assume that a client is depressed about being in the hospital and so may fail to ask him why he seems sad.

During the study process, you can ask yourself how a particular concept is relevant to the application of the nursing process to client care. **Justify** (prove or show to be valid) your ideas to yourself and to another student.

Consistency vs. Inconsistency

Consistency means using principles and concepts appropriately for related applications. For instance, if you are using a particular nursing diagnosis based on accepted indicators, it should be applied when those indicators are present and should not be used when the indicators are not present. Failure to follow this standard results in inconsistent use of the nursing diagnosis.

Consistency can also refer to recognizing and using basic concepts appropriately whenever they apply. For example, knowing the basic actions of epinephrine will enable you to predict client responses to the administration of the drug. It will also help you understand that the client has the same response when an increased secretion of epinephrine is released by the client's kidneys.

Logical vs. Illogical

To be logical means to build one idea upon another so that the conclusion is based on a sequence of steps. Each step should be reasonable and related to the step before it and the step after it. Many symptoms that clients exhibit can be understood logically based on your knowledge of normal physiology and the changes produced by the client's given disease or malady. The successful student will make more efficient use of study time by identifying the logical basis of the material being presented.

The author of a nursing textbook uses nursing logic to organize the content of the book. You must use your own logic to grasp the meaning of the material. Do this by discovering the logic of the author. In this way you will begin to think within the logic of nursing.

Depth vs. Superficiality

Busy students may be tempted to rely on the specific learning objectives and the teacher's pretest review as indicators of the amount of material they must master. This, however, may result in only a superficial understanding of basic processes and principles. Students can improve their ability to recognize the depth to which they must explore concepts and ideas. There is no easy way to do this, but knowing that different material requires different depth of study can assist the student. With time, these decisions will be easier to make. Your instructor and the learning aids within your textbook are useful guides. The more you use them, the better you will become at identifying relevant information and the appropriate depth of knowledge required to make good clinical decisions.

Completeness vs. Incompleteness

During the assessment phase of client care it is important that the nurse know when the client database is sufficient. Proper nursing care is based on identification of priority needs. The nurse will provide care only for those problems that have been identified. Although the physician orders treatments related to the medical diagnosis, these orders are not meant to direct all required care. Nursing care is essential to client well-being. Incomplete information or analysis of client needs will result in inappropriate or inadequate nursing care. Of course, your ability to identify and prioritize client care problems depends on the completeness of your knowledge base. This standard is related to accuracy. An incomplete database leads to inaccurate conclusions.

Significance vs. Triviality

When making decisions or sorting out information it is important for the nurse to identify information that is necessary for good decision making. Being able to recognize irrelevant facts or data that are not helpful for the problem at hand is an important skill. It is easy for a student to view all the material in a textbook as equally significant. Learning to identify significant (important) concepts will minimize the chances of your being distracted by trivial material.

Adequacy vs. Inadequacy

In solving problems or exploring a subject, adequacy refers to the degree to which the available information is sufficient for the purpose and the amount of time and effort spent on the matter. When making clinical decisions, the nurse must be able to recognize when there is sufficient information upon which to base a decision. Premature closure of the process or the inability to decide because of fear that there is not enough information are equally detrimental to quality thinking.

As you study each chapter you will be given information that will help you identify the basic information required to care for each client. Knowing that good client care decisions are based on good preparation by the nurse can help you fit information into the logic of nursing.

Fairness vs. Bias

You, along with other students, come to the educational setting with a set of beliefs, opinions, and points of view. People are predisposed to believe that what they think is true must be true. The improvement of the quality of your thinking depends on your ability to identify the biases present in your thinking and the biases present in the thinking of others. Commitment to fairness will lead a person to challenge conclusions that are based on personal bias. A nursing example would be the assessment of a person in pain. Each individual has learned a way to respond to pain: Some become quiet, some complain loudly, some are stoic, and some are emotional. When a nurse who has a stoic response to pain assesses a person who has an emotional response to pain, it is possible that the nurse will allow personal values to influence the assessment. This can lead to stereotyping of a client as a "cry baby," with the result being that the nurse provides inadequate pain control for the client.

REASONING AND PROBLEM-SOLVING

Reasoning has been defined as the process of figuring things out by using critical thinking skills. Although reasoning involves thinking, all thinking is not reasoning. A human being is thinking when daydreaming, jumping to conclusions, stereotyping, or deciding to listen to music. None of these activities can be called reasoning. In order to use reasoning, to figure things out, or to problem-solve, the student must become familiar with the components of reasoning. These elements are purpose, the question at issue, assumptions, point of view, data and information, concepts, inferences and conclusions, and implications and consequences (Paul & Willsen, 1993). Table 1-4 illustrates the elements of thought in reasoning.

Table 1-4 THE ELEMENTS OF THOUGHT IN REASONING

1. All reasoning has a PURPOSE.
   - Take time to state your purpose clearly
   - Distinguish your purpose from related purposes
   - Check periodically to be sure you are still on target
   - Choose significant and realistic purposes

2. All reasoning is an attempt TO FIGURE SOMETHING OUT, TO SETTLE SOME QUESTION, TO SOLVE SOME PROBLEM.
   - Take time to clearly and simply state the question at issue
   - Express the question in several ways to clarify its meaning and scope
   - Break the question into subquestions
   - Identify whether it is a factual question, a preference question, or a question that requires reasoning

3. All reasoning is based on ASSUMPTIONS.
   - Clearly identify your assumptions and check for their probable validity
   - Check the consistency of your assumptions
   - Reexamine the question at issue when assumptions prove insupportable

4. All reasoning is done from some POINT OF VIEW.
   - Identify your own point of view and its limitations
   - Seek other points of view and identify their strengths as well as their weaknesses
   - Strive to be fairminded in evaluating all points of view

5. All reasoning is based on DATA AND INFORMATION.
   - Restrict your claims to those supported by sufficient data
   - Lay out the evidence clearly
   - Search for information against your position and explain its relevance

6. All reasoning is expressed through, and shaped by, CONCEPTS.
   - Identify each concept that is needed to explore the problem, and precisely define it
   - Explain the choice of important concepts and the implications of each
   - Define when concepts are used vaguely or inappropriately

7. All reasoning contains INFERENCES by which we draw CONCLUSIONS and give meaning to data.
   - Tie inferences tightly and directly from evidence to conclusions
   - Seek inferences that are deep, consistent, and logical
   - Identify the relative strength of each of your inferences

8. All reasoning leads somewhere and has IMPLICATIONS AND CONSEQUENCES.
   - Trace out a variety of implications and consequences that stem from your reasoning
   - Search for negative as well as positive consequences
   - Anticipate unusual or unexpected consequences from various points of view

Courtesy of The Foundation for Critical Thinking, Dillon, CA.

Purpose

All reasoning is directed toward some specific purpose. This is one way whereby reasoning is different from daydreaming. In the case of the nursing student, the purpose of reasoning is to effectively solve client care problems. During your formal education process, you will use reasoning to discover the logic of the practice of nursing.

The Question at Issue

The reasoning process has as its purpose the solution to some problem. This problem must be clearly defined. At the beginning of each study period, you must be able to state clearly the particular problems presented by this particular material. In the clinical setting, good clinical judgment begins with the clear statement of the problems presented by each client. One purpose of the nursing process is to identify client problems in a sufficiently clear and simple manner to enable appropriate responses by the nurse.

Assumptions

Assumptions are those ideas or things that are taken for granted. In the process of reasoning, you must be aware of the assumptions that are made in contrast to the facts that are known. Assumptions are accepted as being true without examination. Assuming certain things may be helpful in problem-solving, but an attempt should be made to recognize the assumptions. An example of an assumption is that nursing makes a difference in the outcome of a client's illness. It is evident that this is a necessary assumption for the nurse to make in order to engage in problem-solving related to client care needs; but it is also important for the nurse to examine this assumption from time to time. One of the issues in nursing today is the question of what nurses do and what preparation is necessary.

It is important to remember that assumptions that have proven reliable can help in decision making. It is just as true that faulty assumptions may cause you to draw faulty conclusions and may lead to poor problem-solving. Learn to recognize your own assumptions and those of others. Never be afraid to challenge your own assumptions or to ask others to clarify the assumptions they are using.

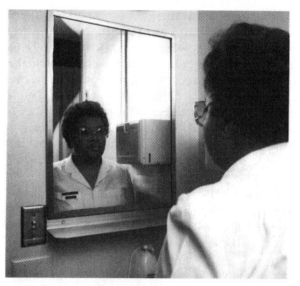

Figure 1-4 To be effective problem-solvers and critical thinkers, nurses must first take a good look at their own ideas and beliefs.

Point of View

Each person reasons using his own logic. Logic consists of previous experience, the quality of thinking already acquired, available information, and many other factors. These factors work together to give each person a unique way of thinking and a unique perspective. This unique perspective determines the individual's point of view. This can be conceptualized by thinking about what a person can see from a small window as compared to a view of the same landscape from an airplane. Each person will see things differently. They may both see a house but each person's view of the house may differ. In the same way, the individual's point of view determines what facts and information will be noticed, the relative importance assigned to each bit of information, and even the acceptable solutions to the problem. You must take the time to recognize your own point of view and to affirm the right of others to have their own points of view (Figure 1-4).

Data and Information

Data and information are the basic materials of reasoning. These are needed in order to define the problem under consideration and to find the solution. During the nursing education program, you may often feel overwhelmed by the quantity of data and information that is presented to you. The result may be that you attempt to practice rote memorization. If data and information are seen as the evidence for reasoning and for problem-solving, however, the process will be more than an exercise in memory. There is a logical relationship between the ideas and facts that compose the content of the nursing course. This logic can be discovered by reasoning. Once the logic is found, the information can be used for problem-solving. Be sure to also look for evidence against your position.

Concepts

The evidence given in support of a conclusion consists of one or more statements relating the conclusion to the problem and to the supporting facts. Reasons must be logically related to the information; in other words, the conclusion cannot be based on something apart from the reasoning process. The concepts (such as pain, adaptation, and so on) that support the nursing process must be part of the evidence supporting a nursing judgment.

Inferences and Conclusions

Reasoning requires interpretation of facts and information. The interpretation must be justifiable in light of the relevant facts. It must be supported by logical connections to the problem and to appropriate data and information. Such interpretation can be called a judgment or inference. Too many times, students state opinions as judgments or inferences. This occurs when interpretations are based on personal preferences rather than on the information that is pertinent to the solution of the problem and on accepted authoritative information.

Properly drawing judgments or inferences is basic to thinking well. An inference results from the following kind of thinking: "Because that is true, then this must be true." For example, you have learned that when the body's temperature goes above normal, the body's metabolic rate increases. You also know that increased metabolism requires more oxygen for the tissues. One way more oxygen can be delivered to the tissues is to increase the heart rate. From these facts, you can infer that an elevated body temperature may result in an increased heart rate.

The product of reasoning is a conclusion in regard to the problem. The conclusion is the answer to the question that began the process. The conclusion must be logical and must

answer the question. It must be based on the proper information and be logically related to the question.

Implications and Consequences

As an outcome of the reasoning process, more than one solution will usually be apparent. At this point, it will be necessary
to examine the implications of each solution. This may require
thinking about the ease with which a solution can be applied,
the ability of a person to carry out the required actions, or the
risks involved.

The outcomes of a particular approach to a problem under
consideration are important. Consequences can result from
action or inaction. Responsible problem-solving requires that all
known consequences be acknowledged. Of course, it is not
possible to predict all consequences; but the possible outcomes
should be examined as completely as possible.

TRAITS OF A DISCIPLINED THINKER

The presentation in this chapter of some of the requirements
of critical thinking will not make anyone think critically. By in-
corporating the idea that thinking about the quality of your own
thinking in relation to UIS is a desirable goal, you can improve
your own thinking. Improved thinking is not something that can
be acquired in a day or two. It is like any high-level skill; it takes
time, effort, and disciplined practice. The result is well worth it,

PROFESSIONAL TIP

Critical Thinking

Critical thinking is far more than an academic exercise. As a
nurse, you are responsible for helping clients achieve and
maintain their optimal level of health. To help sharpen your
critical thinking skills, get in the habit of asking yourself
questions such as "Why is this procedure being done?"
"What are its benefits?" and "Do I see alternatives that might
result in better client outcomes?" Do this several times a day
while caring for clients. Training yourself to think critically
about all client care and interactions will help you to
become a more skilled and compassionate professional.

however. Consistent efforts to improve your thinking can result in the acquisition of the traits of an educated person (Paul & Willsen, 1993). These traits, or habitual ways of thinking, can be recognized by others and can enable a person to compete successfully in the high-tech world.

Reason

The educated person will be reasonable. This simply means that the person values reasoning in himself and in others. This person will not be interested in placing blame or dodging responsibility. There will be a commitment to problem-solving and to cooperative efforts aimed at logically solving the problems encountered in the workplace.

Humility

Another quality that results from consistent efforts to practice disciplined thinking is intellectual humility. To be intellectually humble means that an individual is aware of how much he does not know. There will be a willingness to examine conclusions and beliefs based on new evidence. There will be respect for the thoughts and ideas of others and a sense of continually learning and improving one's own thinking.

Courage

The thinking person will be intellectually courageous. One of the characteristics of this trait is a willingness to take unpopular positions based on reasoning. Conclusions and beliefs that direct activities will thus be the result of disciplined thinking, rather than the opinions of the group.

Integrity

Integrity refers to the constancy of one's actions, meaning that, based on reasoning, the same standards are applied consistently and are not changed to suit circumstances or personal prejudices. The result is a person whose behavior is in harmony with his thinking.

Perseverance

Finally, the thinking person will be capable of intellectual perseverance, meaning a willingness to undertake the challenge of completing hard intellectual tasks. Not giving up, pursuing a solution until its conclusion, and maintaining the quality of thinking are the qualities related to this trait.

CRITICAL THINKING IN NURSING

Alfaro-Lafevre (1999) developed the following description of critical thinking in nursing. Critical thinking in nursing:

- entails purposeful, outcome-directed (results-oriented) thinking.
- is driven by client, family, and community needs.
- is based on principles of nursing process and scientific method.
- requires specific knowledge, skills, and experience.
- is guided by professional standards and ethics codes.
- requires strategies that maximize human potential and compensate for problems created by human nature.
- is constantly reevaluating, self-correcting, and striving to improve.

Nursing Process

The nursing process is a tool to assist in critical thinking when caring for clients. It is dynamic; nurses move back and forth between the steps of the nursing process as is appropriate with each client.

Nursing Standards/Practice Guidelines

National practice standards state how nurses are expected to act when caring for clients. Nursing practice standards, developed by the National Federation of Licensed Practical Nurses (NFLPN), for the LP/VN are found in Appendix A.

Each health care agency develops standards and guidelines to aid in decisions. These may be called protocols, policies, procedures, standards of care, care plans, or critical pathways. Also, the Agency for Healthcare Research and Quality (AHRQ) has developed clinical practice guidelines for 19 specific problems. Included in these guidelines are ones for acute pain management, cancer pain, depression, pressure ulcers, low-back problems, and urinary incontinence.

The nursing process and practice guidelines are tools to assist the nurse in making client care decisions. Critical thinking must be used to recognize when a client situation differs from the guidelines. Guidelines are not to be followed blindly.

CASE STUDY

This activity is designed to give you an opportunity to apply the knowledge and skills you have gained. This means that you will be expected to use critical thinking skills as you explore selected nursing situations. For this chapter, the scenario is to be written by you and about you.

1. Review the four basic skills of critical thinking: reading, writing, listening, and speaking.

2. Identify specifically the precise skills you want to improve. Write in your own words what you want to accomplish in terms of positive skills you will possess when you have implemented your plan and accomplished your goal. This means that you will identify both specific performance measures for your reading, writing, speaking, and listening skills, and time frames for points at which you will evaluate your performance. For example, if you set a goal of being able to identify the main points of an assigned reading, how would you measure that? In comparison with others in your study group? By your test performance? Write down your evaluation criteria and the time frames for evaluation.

3. When you have clearly stated in writing which basic skills you will work on, review the material in this chapter or from other resources to identify possible ways to work on those skills. Choose the most appropriate methods for you. Write down your plan. Be precise and specific.

4. Your next step is to actually put your plan into action by doing what you have planned to do.

5. Evaluate your actions to see whether they have resulted in the desired outcome. In order to perform a valid evaluation, you must evaluate your performance based on the evaluation criteria and goals you outlined in number 2.

continues

Case Study *continued*

6. Realize that you must know yourself well. If the processes of critical thinking and reasoning are new to you, select only one or two things on which to work. If you feel more adventurous, use the suggested process to explore your thinking in relation to the universal standards of thought and to the traits of a thoughtful person. Assess your problem-solving style in relation to the elements of thought in reasoning.

SUMMARY

- Critical thinking is a disciplined way of thinking that the nursing student can begin to develop. The effective use of the nursing process depends on the ability to think well.
- There are many ways to define critical thinking. Essential components of any definition should emphasize self-assessment of the quality of one's own thinking according to standards of excellence and careful use of the elements of reasoning.
- Four basic intellectual skills are essential to quality thinking: critical reading, critical listening, critical writing, and critical speaking.
- The spectrum of Universal Intellectual Standards (UIS) can be the measure of competence in each of the basic skills.
- Reasoning is the process of applying critical thinking to some problem so as to find an answer or to figure something out. Therefore, reasoning has a purpose. The process of reasoning requires that attention be paid to the elements of thought in reasoning and to the UIS.
- When students begin to be aware of their own thinking and begin to assume responsibility for it, they will begin to use their own logic to discover the logic of nursing. The result will be better learning and the ability to make high-quality decisions related to client care.
- Consistent attention to improving the quality of thinking will produce the traits of an educated nurse. The student will become intellectually reasonable, humble, and courageous and will possess intellectual integrity and perseverance.

Review Questions

1. A branch of learning or field of study is called a:
   a. career.
   b. movement.
   c. principle.
   d. discipline.

2. Fundamental to quality thinking is the ability to think:
   a. clearly.
   b. effectively.
   c. quantitatively.
   d. with ambiguity.

3. The person who is concrete or exact when stating or applying a fact is practicing the standard for critical thinking called:
   a. accuracy.
   b. precision.
   c. consistency.
   d. specificity.

4. The person who has the ability to separate needed information from information not needed at the present time is practicing the standard for critical thinking called:
   a. logic.
   b. relevance.
   c. adequacy.
   d. significance.

5. Ideas or things that are taken for granted are called:
   a. evidences.
   b. inferences.
   c. assumptions.
   d. implications.

6. The person who is willing to take an unpopular position based on reasoning is said to have:
   a. courage.
   b. humility.
   c. integrity.
   d. perseverance.

Key Terms

Match the following terms with their correct definitions.

___ 1. Concept

___ 2. Critical
    Thinking

___ 3. Discipline

___ 4. Disciplined

___ 5. Judgment

___ 6. Justify

___ 7. Logic

___ 8. Opinion

___ 9. Reasoning

___ 10. Reflective

___ 11. Standard

a. To prove or show to be valid.
b. Use of the elements of thought to solve a problem or settle a question.
c. Mode of thinking—about any subject, content, or problem— whereby the thinker improves the quality of her thinking by skillfully taking charge of the structures inherent in thinking and imposing intellectual standards (or a level of degree of quality) upon them.
d. Branch of learning, field of study, or occupation requiring specialized knowledge.
e. Level or degree of quality.
f. Mental picture of abstract phenomena that serves to organize observations related to that phenomena.
g. Trained by instruction and exercise.
h. Formal principles of a branch of knowledge (such as nursing).
i. Introspective.
j. Conclusions that are based on sound reasoning and can be supported by evidence.
k. Subjective belief.

Abbreviation Review

Write the meaning or definition of the following abbreviations, acronyms, and symbols.

1. UIS _____

Exercises and Activities

1. Complete the following statements.
   a. To use the nursing process effectively, you must develop the skills of _____.
   b. Subjective beliefs are called _____.
   c. Conclusions based on sound reasoning and supported by evidence are _____.
   d. Ideas or things taken for granted are called _____.
   e. The traits of a disciplined thinker include _____.
   f. The nursing process is the application of _____ to the practice of nursing.
   g. A person's _____ is based on many factors that combine to develop a unique way of thinking and a unique perspective.
   h. To _____ an idea is to prove it or show it to be valid.
   i. The _____ (or UIS) lists criteria for determining the quality of thinking skills.
   j. The answer to a question that began a process of reasoning is called a _____.

2. The process of critical thinking is based on developing the following four skills: critical reading, critical listening, critical writing, and critical speaking.
   a. List three tactics that will help you develop critical reading skills.
      (1) _____
      (2) _____
      (3) _____
   b. Write two questions that you can ask yourself to support critical listening skills.
      (1) _____
      (2) _____
   c. List three critical writing techniques that improve the ability to state your thoughts clearly.
      (1) _____
      (2) _____
      (3) _____
   d. Give three actions that should be avoided in critical speaking.
      (1) _____
      (2) _____
      (3) _____

3. Read the following paragraph:

   Greed and waste have been identified as major problems of the U.S. health care system. Whether these
   problems are caused by defensive practice, consumer
   demand, or professional economics is irrelevant to
   the public. Success in reform depends on starting
   where the public expects reform should begin: elimi-
   nating the greed of providers and the waste in the
   health care system. Further, people in the United
   States have become suspicious of health care
   providers. The high level of esteem in which medicine has traditionally been held has eroded over the
   past few years. Consumers, increasingly tired of pay-
   ing the high cost of care, are questioning medical
   practices and fees. However, the public is not dis-
   illusioned with nurses. This positive perception of
   nurses will be important as patterns of reform are
   established.

   a. What is the question at issue in this paragraph?

   _____

   _____

   b. What assumptions may have been stated here?

   _____

   _____

   c. Does this writing show a point of view?

   _____

   _____

   d. List the concepts that you see in the paragraph.

   _____

   _____

   e. What inferences and conclusions have been drawn?

   _____

   _____

   f. Has the writer discussed implications or consequences?

   _____

   _____

   g. Are there any words that could have been misunderstood that might affect the paragraph's clarity?

   _____

   _____

Self-Assessment Questions

Circle the letter that corresponds to the best answer for each question.

1. All reasoning is based on using the skills of:
    a. critical thinking.
    b. decision making.
    c. concept formation.
    d. inferences.

2. Anyone can work toward becoming a better thinker by developing:
    a. introspective thinking techniques.
    b. opinions based on sound reasoning.
    c. specific attitudes, traits, and skills.
    d. philosophy statements related to nursing.

3. Students may improve their critical listening skills by:
    a. requesting a bibliography.
    b. taking word-for-word notes.
    c. focusing on the mannerisms of the speaker.
    d. carrying on a mental dialogue with the speaker.

4. All reasoning is an attempt to:
    a. problem-solve.
    b. define concepts.
    c. determine assumptions.
    d. develop personal values.

5. Which statement is an example of an assumption?
    a. The minority population of the United States is growing every year.
    b. Women are better caretakers of children than are men.
    c. Clients want to be comfortable and free of pain.
    d. Elderly clients are better off at home.

6. A client wants to go home early from the hospital, saying, "My family can take better care of me at home than you can here." It is most important for the nurse to consider:
    a. her personal biases.
    b. the patient's diagnosis.
    c. home health care nursing.
    d. the implications or consequences.

7. A nurse evaluates a client as overreacting to pain based on her own reaction to pain. This would be an example of:

   a. reasoning.
   b. personal bias.
   c. an inference.
   d. empathy.

WEB FLASH!

- Search the web for sites dealing with critical thinking. What date is the oldest entry? What date is the newest entry?
- Search the web using the names of the major nursing organizations such as National Federation of Licensed Practical Nurses (NFLPN), National Association of Practical Nurse Education and Service, Inc. (NAPNES), and the National League for Nursing (NLN). Do they have web sites that include pages that might offer information on critical thinking? What about nursing standards or practice guidelines?

Critical Thinking Questions

1. Of the four basic skills of critical thinking, which one are you able to do best? Why? How do you know?

2. How do you take responsibility for your own thinking?

References/Suggested Readings

Alfaro-LeFevre, R. (1999). *Critical thinking in nursing: A practical approach* (2nd ed.). Philadelphia: W. B. Saunders Company.

Baker, C. R. (1996). Reflective learning: A teaching strategy for critical thinking. *Journal of Nursing Education, 35*, 19–22.

Birx, E. (1993). Critical thinking and theory-based practice. *Holistic Nursing Practice, 7*(3).

Boucher, M. (1998). Delegation alert! *AJN, 98*(2), 26–32.

Brigham, C. (1993). Nursing education and critical thinking: Interplay of content and thinking. *Holistic Nursing Practice, 7*(3).

Brookfield, S. (1993). On impostership, cultural suicide and owners dangers: How nurses learn critical thinking. *Journal of Continuing Education in Nursing, 24*(5), 179–205.

Center for Critical Thinking. (1997). *Critical thinking in living, working & learning (a real time video)* [On-line]. Available: www.uncp.edu/home/vanderhoof/criticalthinking.ram

Center for Critical Thinking. (2000, January 25). *A brief history of the idea of critical thinking* [On-line]. Available: http://www.critical thinking.org/University/univlibrary/cthistory.nclk

Center for Critical Thinking. (2000, January 25). *Valuable intellectual traits* [On-line]. Available: www.criticalthinking.org/University/univlibrary/intraits.nclk

Chaffee, J. (1998). *The thinker's way.* Boston: Little, Brown and Company.

Chaffee, J. (1999). *The thinker's guide to college success.* Boston: Houghton Mifflin Company.

Chaffee, J. (2000). *Thinking critically* (6th ed.). Boston: Houghton Mifflin College.

Conger, M., & Mezza, I. (1996). Fostering critical thinking in nursing students in the clinical setting. *Nurse Educator, 21*(3), 11–15.

Dossey, B., & Dossey, L. (1998). Body-mind-spirit: Attending to holistic care. *AJN, 98*(8), 35–38.

Elder, L., & Paul, R. (2000, January 25). *Universal intellectual standards* [On-line]. Available: www.criticalthinking.org/University.univlibrary/unistan.nclk

Ennis, R. H. (1985). A logical basis for measuring critical thinking skills. *Educational Leadership, 43*, 44–48.

Eskreis, T. (1998). Seven common legal pitfalls in nursing. *AJN, 98*(4), 34–41.

Facioñe, N. (2000). *Critical thinking assessment in nursing education programs: An aggregate data analysis.* Millbrae, CA: California Academic Press.

Fonteyn, M. (1998). *Thinking strategies for nursing practice.* Philadelphia: Lippincott Williams & Wilkins.

Guffey, M. E. (1998). *Five steps to better critical thinking, problem-solving and decision-making skills* [On-line]. Available: www.westwords.com/GUFFEY/critical.html

Heaslip, P. (1993, September). Intellectual standards: What are they? *Critical Connections* [Newsletter of the Critical Thinking Interest Group, University College of the Cariboo, Kamloops, B.C.]

Heaslip, P. (1994, November). *Defining critical thinking. Dialogue: A Critical Thinking Newsletter for Nurses, 3.*

Kurfiss, J. (1988). *Critical thinking: Theory, research, practice and possibilities.* Washington, DC: Association for the Study of Higher Education. (ASHE-ERIC Higher Education Report No. 2)

Lashley, M., & Wittstadt, R. (1993). Writing across the curriculum: An integrated curricular approach to developing critical thinking through writing. *Journal of Nursing Education, 32*(9), 422–424.

Miller, M., & Babcock, D. (1996). *Critical thinking applied to nursing.* St. Louis, MO: Mosby-Year Book.

Miller, M. A., & Malcolm, N. S. (1990). Critical thinking in the nursing curriculum. *Nursing & Health Care, 11,* 66–73.

Norris, S. P., & Ennis, R. H. (1989). *Evaluating critical thinking.* Pacific Grove, CA: Midwest Publication.

Paul, R. (1990). *Critical thinking: What every person needs to survive in a rapidly changing world.* Rohnert Park, CA: Center for Critical Thinking and Moral Critique, Sonoma State University.

Paul, R. (1993). *Critical thinking: How to prepare students for a rapidly changing world.* Santa Rosa, CA: Foundation for Critical Thinking.

Paul, R., & Elder, L. (2000, January 25). *Helping students assess their thinking* [On-line]. Available: www.criticalthinking.org/University/univlibrary/helps.nclk

Paul, R., & Elder, L. (2000). *Critical thinking: Tools for taking charge of your learning and your life.* Upper Saddle River, NJ: Prentice Hall.

Paul, R., & Willsen, J. (1993). *Critical thinking from an ideal evolves an imperative.* Santa Rosa, CA: The Foundation for Critical Thinking.

Ruggiero, V. (2000). *The art of thinking: A guide to critical and creative thought* (6th ed.). New York: Longman.

Saucier, B., Stevens, K., & Williams, G. (2000). Critical thinking outcomes of computer-assisted instruction versus written nursing process. *Nursing and Health Care Perspectives, 21*(5), 240–246.

Scriven, M., & Paul, R. (1996). *Defining critical thinking* [On-line]. (Center for Critical Thinking at Sonoma State University, Rohnert Park, CA.) Available: http://www.criticalthinking.org/University/univclass/defining.nclk

Wilkinson, J. (1996). *Nursing process: A critical thinking approach* (2nd ed.). Menlo Park, CA: Addison-Wesley.

Worrell, P. J. (1990). Metacognition: Implications for instruction in nursing education. *Journal of Nursing Education, 29*(4), 170–175.

Resources

California Academic Press, 217 La Cruz Avenue, Millbrae, CA 94030, 650-697-5628, www.calpress.com/, email: info@calpress.com

Center for Critical Thinking at Sonoma State University, Box 220, Dillon Beach, CA 94929, 707-878-9100, www.criticalthinking.org

Foundation for Critical Thinking, P.O. Box 220, Dillon Beach, CA 94929, 800-833-3645

International Center for the Assessment of Higher Order Thinking (ICAT), 707-878-9100, http://www.criticalthinking.org/icat.nclk

National Council for Excellence in Critical Thinking, P.O. Box 220, Dillon Beach, CA 94929, 707-878-9100, www.criticalthinking.org/ncect.nclk

SKILLS FOR SUCCESS

LEARNING OBJECTIVES

Upon completion of this chapter, you should be able to:
- *Define key terms.*
- *Outline strategies for developing a positive attitude toward the learner role.*
- *Identify strategies for developing proficiency in basic skills.*
- *Identify learning-style methods that can be incorporated for effective study.*
- *Design a time-management plan.*
- *Design a personal study plan.*
- *Identify strategies for improving test-taking outcomes.*
- *Complete a stress-reduction exercise using guided imagery.*

KEY TERMS

ability	learning	perfectionism
anxiety	learning disability	procrastination
attitude	learning style	time management
attribute	metacognition	
encoding	mnemonics	

INTRODUCTION

Learning is defined as the act or process of acquiring knowledge and/or skill in a particular subject. An individual never stops learning. This is especially true in the field of nursing and health care. The amount of information within the health care

PROFESSIONAL TIP

Learning
The key to your success is not how you will be taught, but how you decide to learn.

domain has expanded exponentially in just the past several years. Consider, for example, the advances in drug therapies, complementary alternative therapies, and genetics. By graduation, some of the information learned in the beginning of the program will have been displaced by new information and discoveries. We are living in the information age and have constant access to thousands of pieces of information through various media, including television and the Internet. Knowledge is never static. Learning, defined as the act of acquiring knowledge, is also not static, but, rather, is a lifelong process.

Individuals seek knowledge to effect some type of change. As a student, you are seeking knowledge to learn skills and to prepare yourself for a career in nursing. Referring to yourself as a learner implies that you are an active participant in the learning process, as opposed to a passive recipient of information. You bring to this new adventure yourself, your past experiences, your abilities, and your motivation to master the knowledge necessary to reach your goals. You have already learned much in your lifetime and are ready to continue the process. It is important that you take some time to think about the competencies needed for the role of learner. It is equally important that you realize that *you* are in charge of developing the competencies that will enable you to learn.

The learning you are seeking will afford you the knowledge and skills necessary to become a nurse and, thus, to demonstrate your ability to competently provide care to clients who seek your professional talents. Nursing education is different from many other college majors in the turnaround time allowed for learning. Few other disciplines require the student to apply on Thursday that which was acquired on Monday. Nursing students must acquire a greater depth of understanding in a shorter amount of time; to achieve this, basic learning processes will need to be well developed.

This chapter addresses *how* you learn rather than *what* you learn. It focuses on competencies necessary to master the learning process: attitude, basic skills, learning style, time management, study strategies, critical thinking, and test-taking strategies. Assessing which habits you already practice and which ones you have yet to incorporate, internalize, and utilize will assist you in improving your process of learning. As you do so, your potential for attaining your goals will increase.

DEVELOP A POSITIVE ATTITUDE

Attitude is defined as a manner, feeling, or position toward a person or thing. In order to effect change in your behavior, you must first develop a positive attitude about this experience you are about to begin. You are in charge of setting yourself up for success. This is your opportunity to acquire the knowledge and skills that will make it possible for you to reach the goal of becoming a licensed practical/vocational nurse. You must develop a positive attitude toward yourself as a person and a learner, as well as a genuine desire to learn. To maintain this attitude late at night when you are struggling over the names of the latest drugs and writing client assessments, you must be convinced that you have the capability to complete your task, that some intrinsic factor will be able to support you in the pursuit of your goal. This positive self-attitude sustains the question "Why am I doing this?" Among the strategies you can practice to help you build a positive attitude are the following:

- Create positive self-images, and visualize yourself attaining your goals.
- Recognize your abilities.
- Identify realistic expectations.

Create Positive Self-Images

To begin to create a positive self-image, you must know those attributes that are unique to you. An **attribute** is a characteristic, either positive or negative, that belongs to you. For instance, some positive attributes that are typical to nurses include caring and compassion. Attributes are sometimes referred to as strengths and weaknesses. Whatever you call them, you must actively engage in listing and recalling these qualities about yourself. Using a chart like the one presented in Figure 2-1, list as many words describing your attributes as you can. List both positive and negative qualities.

My attribute chart	
Positive Attributes	Negative Attributes

Figure 2-1 Attribute Chart

Which side has more entries? Did you start with the negative list? It is unfortunate that sometimes we can recall the negatives faster than the positives. We often speak about ourselves in negative terms, which creates negative self-images. For example, you may recall thinking some of the following: "I wish I were thinner . . . ," "I hope I can do this, I'm not very good at math." Neither of these statements draws a positive image of the speaker. You may need to lose 10 pounds, or improve your math skills, but these are not the total measure of your attributes. If they are the only qualities you recall, they might become the overall image you see of yourself. Regardless of where you started, you must concentrate on the positive side of the chart. You must actively recall your positive side at least as often as you recount the things that could be improved.

Begin to speak of yourself in positive terms and accept compliments from yourself! You will be building the sustenance to get through the rough parts of the new role you have taken on. When an assignment is particularly difficult you can refocus from "I hope I can do this. I have never been good at math" to "I can read and follow the chapter instructions on how to complete the problems." This simple restatement can sometimes make the difference in whether we succeed or fail at our attempts to acquire new knowledge.

The list does not have to stop at just the words you write today. Continue to practice and do periodic self-assessments. You will add more and more words to the positive side and begin to compliment yourself more often. When things go awry you will be able to draw on these positive attributes and know that you have these strengths.

Recognize Your Abilities

Recognizing your abilities is also an attitude builder. **Ability** can be defined as competence in an activity. An ability is something you can learn; competency is proficiency in a task. Your degree of competence as a nurse will depend on such factors as prior exposure, motivation, how often and with whom you practice, expectations of those things that you should be doing, and a willingness to laugh at attempts and learn from mistakes.

You have abilities and skills that you perform well. To acquire these things took courage, discipline, and hard work. Recalling these abilities and the ways you developed competency in them not only adds to your positive self-image, but showcases your strengths. Begin to practice recalling your abilities by completing the exercise described in Figure 2-2. Under each of the columns (A and B), write an ending to each statement and place it in the big box. Next, list all of the skills you need to be able to be "really good" at that task. Write these skills in the smaller boxes. Do not worry if you cannot fill all the small boxes or if you run out of boxes.

As an example for column A, maybe you wrote, "I am really good at cooking." Following are some skills you could have included in the smaller boxes:

- *Arithmetic:* You must have an understanding of fractions and the relationships of parts to the whole.
- *Reading:* You must comprehend the words in the recipe in order to follow all the steps.
- *Prioritizing:* You must know with what to start in order to have all of the food ready at the same time.
- *Risk taker:* You may worry about whether your guests will like your dish, but you persist, confident in your ability to turn the raw ingredients into a delicious meal.

Now look at column B, using math as an example. Mathematics is an ability you must develop in order to safely

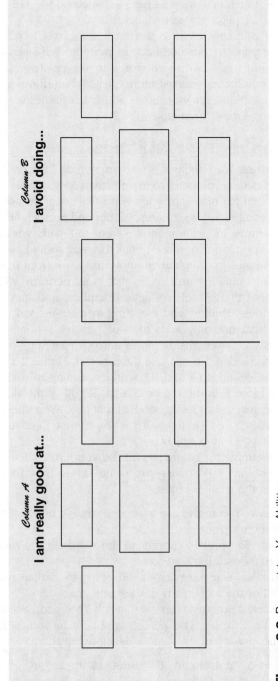

Figure 2-2 Recognizing Your Abilities

administer medications to your clients. If you view this skill only as something to avoid, you start out with a negative attitude toward an ability you will need. You are creating a negative image of yourself completing this task. Instead, look to your past experiences for your strengths; you may realize that you already possess much of the mathematical knowledge you need to correctly compute medication dosages. Realizing this puts a positive slant on this ability.

Now you must develop mathematical competency. Begin by asking yourself which skills are needed to perform mathematical operations. You must pay attention to details, understand the way parts relate to the whole, and have solid skills in arithmetic (addition, subtraction, division, and multiplication). Mathematics requires you to choose appropriate formulas to solve a variety of real-world problems. For example, to give the correct dose of medication to your client, you must know the correct formula to use for the calculation. This is a real-world problem for which you must both choose the correct formula and understand it. You must then accurately perform the arithmetic operations.

Identify Realistic Expectations

As mentioned earlier, developing a positive self-image is of primary importance to learning. Your expectations regarding how you will perform in the role as a learner will affect your attitude toward both yourself and learning. You have an expectation about the way you will progress through this program. Ideally, you will attend all classes, pass all exams, and graduate. Further, your current life responsibilities will cooperate with and support this plan. You will likely, however, encounter at least some obstacles. When you hit that first "speed bump" to your plan, your ability to look at the reality of your expectations will be important in regaining a positive focus. Consider the following example:

> Marissa is a 25-year-old enrolled full time in a nursing program for the fall. She did well in high school and has already attended a college part time prior to this program. Marissa expects that she will get grades in the B and A range, as she did in prior course work. She works full time and has a 4-year-old daughter. When the class schedule is published, the times conflict with one of the days that she works. This will cause her to be 20 minutes late to work on that day. She has not shared with her employer

that she is attending school. She has child care for her daughter, but the need to arrive at the clinical site at 7 A.M. means that she must rearrange her child care and that she will be 30 minutes late for clinical on Fridays. She does not tell her instructors of her time constraints for child care. She has always needed quiet time for study and is a morning person. Marissa finds her reading assignments take twice as long as she had planned. With all her other responsibilities, her only time for study is after her daughter goes to bed. She has a family who lives close by, but she does not like to burden them with baby-sitting. She has always found a way to do things on her own in the past.

Marissa is a capable person, but her expectation of being able to control all the various facets of her life in perfect harmony is unrealistic. Maintaining a positive attitude while in the midst of the stress of completing all the tasks at hand is difficult if not impossible, and the plan is often abandoned. In Marissa's case, abandoning the plan may mean abandoning her plans for school. Marissa's reality is that she cannot increase her time commitment by 30 hours of school work and keep everything else she does at the same level. She must set priorities with regard to the demands on her time, and she must identify realistic expectations for those things that she can accomplish.

When you cannot complete everything on your "to do" list, change the way you approach the list and realign your expectations. One way to do this is to ask for help. Asking for help is not a weakness, it is a success strategy. The most successful people are typically those who know when to ask for help and who have devised a plan to structure that help. In the previous example, Marissa needed to remove some of the stress related to both work and school commitments by informing her supervisor and instructors of her situation and asking for their help in guiding her to manage her many demands. Help may mean something as simple as talking to your instructors so that they know you must leave on Thursdays at 3 P.M., due to work commitments. Present a proactive plan of how you will get the notes and make up the time and then ask them to accommodate you.

If you do not set realistic expectations for yourself, you may fall victim to a positive attitude's biggest enemy, perfectionism. **Perfectionism** is not synonymous with excellence, but rather is an overwhelming expectation of being able to get everything done. This is setting yourself up for failure, as it is a standard no

Table 2-1 BEHAVIORS OF PERFECTIONISTS AND PURSUERS OF EXCELLENCE

PERFECTIONISTS	PURSUERS OF EXCELLENCE
• Reach for impossible goals	• Enjoy meeting high standards within reach
• Value themselves for what they do	• Value themselves for who they are
• Get depressed and give up	• Experience disappointment but keep going
• Are devastated by failure	• Learn from failure
• Remember mistakes and dwell on them	• Correct mistakes, then learn from them
• Can only live with being number one	• Are pleased with knowing they did their best
• Hate criticism	• Welcome criticism
• Have to win to maintain high self-esteem	• Do not have to win to maintain high self-esteem

one can live up to. Table 2-1 suggests some behaviors of perfectionists versus those of pursuers of excellence. Which list describes you most accurately? Remember to strive to be as realistic with your expectations as possible; be patient with yourself and ask for help when needed.

DEVELOP YOUR BASIC SKILLS

Dirkx and Prenger (1997) list the following skills as basic for success in academics and life: reading, arithmetic and mathematics, writing, listening, and speaking. They further describe each of the skills in terms of characteristics that provide a sense of what is expected from the learner in each area (Table 2-2).

When you consider these characteristics, the basic skills do not seem so basic but, rather, take on a new importance. Look at the list and make a quick note of your strengths and weaknesses. You must have a strong foundation in these basic skills to advance your knowledge beyond the level of memorization. You must advance your knowledge level from memorization to comprehension and application. If you are struggling with these basic skills, you will have difficulty advancing. Developing these skills is basic to the habits of successful learners.

Table 2-2 BASIC SKILL COMPETENCY LIST

SKILL	BASIC COMPETENCY
Reading	Locate, understand, and interpret written information in prose and documents, including manuals, graphs, and schedules, to perform tasks; learn from a text by determining the main idea or essential message; identify relevant details, facts, and specifications; infer or locate the meaning of unknown or technical vocabulary; judge the accuracy, appropriateness, style, and plausibility of reports, proposals, or theories from other writers.
Arithmetic and mathematics	Perform basic computations; use basic numerical concepts such as whole numbers and percentages (fractions, decimals) in practical situations; approach practical problems by choosing appropriately from a variety of mathematical techniques.
Writing	Communicate thoughts, ideas, information, and messages; record information completely and accurately; compose and create documents and use language, style, organization, and format appropriate to the subject matter, purpose, and audience; include supporting documentation; attend to detail and check, edit, and revise for correct information, appropriate emphasis, form, grammar, spelling, and punctuation.
Listening	Receive, attend to, interpret, and respond to verbal messages and other cues, such as body language, in ways that are appropriate to the purpose in order to comprehend, learn, evaluate critically, appreciate, or support the speaker.
Speaking	Organize ideas and communicate oral messages appropriate to listeners and situations; use verbal language and other cues such as body language appropriate in style, tone, and level of complexity to the audience and occasion; speak clearly and communicate a message; understand and respond to listener feedback and ask questions when needed.

Adapted from Planning and Implementing Instruction for Adults *(pp. 133–134), by J. Dirkx and S. Prenger, 1997, San Francisco: Jossey-Bass. Copyright 1997 by Jossey-Bass.*

Reading

Ninety percent of your program is in written format. To study effectively, you must be highly adept in the basic skill of reading. Among the several strategies you can effectively implement in your reading and study plan to improve this skill are vocab-

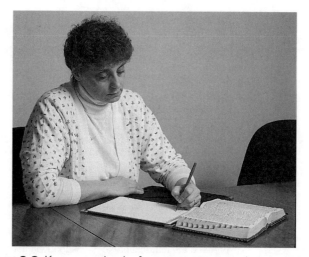

Figure 2-3 Keep a notebook of new terms to expand your vocabulary. Review your notebook and try to use the words in practice daily.

ulary building, comprehension, and reading level. Your basic skill of reading encompasses vocabulary building, which includes the skill of identification and understanding of both English and medical terminology. Investing in quality medical and English dictionaries is a good step to understanding both these languages. Another strategy is simply to take the time when reading to look up the words you do not know (Figure 2-3).

The primary reason for building a strong medical vocabulary is that words are the tools for thinking about and understanding your world, and you are entering the new world of nursing: You must therefore take the time to learn its language. Developing the habit of vocabulary building takes time initially, but as you persist in practicing this skill, your comprehension of the material will increase.

Comprehension goes beyond rote memorization. One sign of true comprehension is the ability to summarize the writer's message. When you summarize, you must recite the material in your own words (Sotiriou & Phillips, 1999). Unless you understand the words you have read, you will not be able to advance your level of knowledge from rote memorization to comprehension. When you are actively reading your nursing textbook and you realize that you are not understanding what you have read, you may find it helpful to use one, some, or all of the five strategies outlined in Table 2-3.

Table 2-3 STRATEGIES TO IMPROVE COMPREHENSION

STRATEGY	EXPLANATION
Reread	Do this after reading one section of the text, or even after one paragraph.
Define new words	Write the definitions of each new word in the margin of your text and then reread the paragraph. Use a small notebook to build your own glossary. Make your own flashcards for further study.
Visualize	Create mental pictures of the material you are reading. You may even want to draw a simple stick figure, and as you continue to read, adjust the picture.
Research	Many times the reason you are unable to comprehend the material presented is that you have insufficient background in the subject. A solution may be to consult another text that is specific to that knowledge base. Use a dictionary, anatomy and physiology text, general subject text (like a psychology text) or a nursing journal to increase your background knowledge in a subject area (Meltzer & Marcus-Palau, 1997).
Summarize	Use your own words to "tell" yourself what you just read and how this connects to what you are going to be doing. Ask yourself, "Why might I need to know this material?"

Reading level is another element of your reading skills. Reading level is not related to what you can understand, but, rather, refers to the length of the words and the sentences used in a text to explain, describe, and convey information. It does not have anything to do with your intelligence, but it has a great deal to do with the length of time it takes you to read.

Arithmetic and Mathematics

The next skill you must develop competency in is that of arithmetic and mathematics. You will be responsible for correctly calculating dosages and safely administering medications to your clients. You must therefore be able to recognize whether your calculations are correct and, upon looking at the amount on a medication order, estimate whether your answer is logical and correct. In nursing, your mastery of mathematical basic skills cannot be overemphasized. Consider the following excerpt from a study of medication errors done in 1998 at a tertiary care teaching hospital; this excerpt underscores the importance of mathematical competency among nurses.

Forty-two percent of dosage errors were considered to put the patient at risk for a serious or severe preventable adverse outcome. Errors in decimal point placement, mathematical calculation, or expression of dosage regime accounted for 59.5% of the dosage errors. The dosage equation was wrong in 29.5% (Lesar, 1998).

Give yourself a reality check on your competency in mathematics and commit to improving those areas where you are weakest. You may want to investigate a resource such as the learning services center at your school, enlist the assistance of a tutor, or use a programmed-learning text to refresh your skills. There are also numerous texts written to assist nursing students in developing these essential skills. Consider also using computer-assisted instruction (CAI) programs or self-paced study modules to hone these skills. Whatever means you use, an honest assessment of your competency in mathematics and a commitment to improvement is essential to your practice in the profession.

Writing

In your role as a student and as a professional, you will need writing skills. Contrary to popular opinion, the influx of the computer into health care has not removed the need for this skill (Figure 2-4). You will be writing client assessments, transfer summaries, discharge summaries, and client-teaching plans, as well as contributing to development of policies and, possibly, even publishing your experiences in a journal. The skill of writing can be practiced and improved. Follow the steps outlined in Table 2-4 as a checklist for your writing assignments.

Listening

The old saying " I know you can hear me, but are you listening?" can be applied to all of us. You must be listening, understanding, and processing information, as opposed to just hearing, when you are in class, as well as when you begin working with clients. When listening during any lecture or demonstration, you receive, interpret, and respond to verbal messages and other cues such as body language. You are attempting to both comprehend the information and evaluate

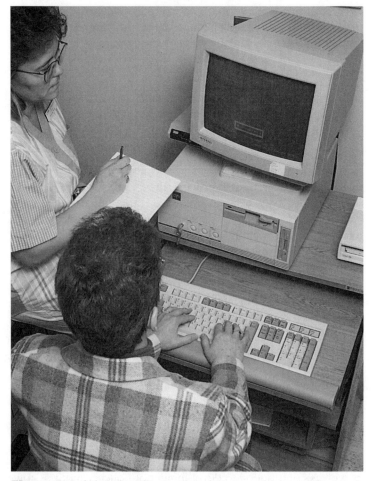

Figure 2-4 Although computers are being used more and more in health care, they do not replace the need for competent writing skills.

the speaker. You may need to polish up on ways that you can improve listening and evaluation skills to make the most of your class time. Class time is a time for listening. Listening effectively can make efficient use of this time to increase your comprehension of the content.

Among the many strategies that can be used to improve listening skills are the following:

- *Being interested in the subject.* Make a connection with the reason you are going to this lecture. What is the connection between the information and your need for the information?

Have you prescanned the information and come with questions about the subject that tie in to how you will use the information presented?

- *Being open to the information.* When you hear a topic and immediately react with your instinct, you often miss the point and some aspect of the presentation you did not consider before. Listening does not automatically mean you will change your mind on topics, but it will allow you to evaluate and incorporate those aspects that are beneficial to you.

- *Not being critical of the speaker.* Focus on the message, not the messenger. The speaker is not there as a member of a theatrical company to entertain you. The speaker's role is to impart information. It is up to you to concentrate on the information that you need to know and apply it properly.

Table 2-4 STEPS TO CLEAR WRITING

STEP	EXPLANATION
Prewrite	Select a subject, collect details about that subject, and develop your writing plan.
Establish a writing plan	Answer the following questions in outline form: • *What* are you writing (essay, test, questionnaire, dialogue)? • *Why* are you writing (to persuade, describe, explain, and narrate)? • *For whom* are you writing (peers, instructors, colleagues)? • *How* are you writing (alone, with a classmate, in a group, on computer)? • *Where* are you writing (on the bus, in the library, at the computer lab)? • *When* will you be writing (consider the time frame for this writing project)?
Write first draft	Organize your writing plan ideas into phrases, sentences, and paragraphs as appropriate to the task, content, and audience. Obtain feedback from your intended audience as to the accuracy, relevance, and understandability of your materials.
Revise	Make changes to improve your writing so it conveys your main idea and purpose.
Edit	Examine critically for errors in spelling, punctuation, grammar, or style.

Adapted from Learning Strategies for Allied Health Students, *by S. Palau and M. Meltzer, 1998, Philadelphia: W. B. Saunders. Copyright 1998 by W. B. Saunders.*

- *Concentrating on the information.* Be present to the lecture. If you find yourself falling asleep, do muscle flexes or breathe deeply to try to stay alert and aware. Imagine test questions that might be asked on the information.
- *Evaluating the information.* Not every word is critical. Relate the information to what you know, where you may use it, and whether you agree with what is said. If you have difficulty with what is being said, use the next strategy to maintain your concentration.
- *Writing down questions as you listen.* This allows you to follow the speaker to the end of her thoughts. Many of your questions may be answered. If not, you have them written down and can refer later to the list. This promotes concentration on the information presented. You will not be distracted trying to remember questions you wanted to ask.

Speaking

Learning to speak or present in front of a group is one of the most-feared activities of many students. Yet as a nurse, you have entered one of the most "speaking"-oriented professions. You will communicate daily with your clients, their families, instructors, peers, ancillary staff members, and the multiple members of the health care team. Learning to do this well will free you

PROFESSIONAL TIP

Speaking

Thorough preparation is an important strategy for speaking about anything. Formulating multiple examples is one way of increasing your comfort level with the given information. For example, if you are asked to explain the way the pancreas produces insulin, you might draw the organ and indicate where the islets of Langerhans are. Or you may use a lock and key to explain the way insulin works to open the channels for glucose to enter the cells. You may trace a cracker as it travels through the body from teeth to cells and indicate just where and when insulin is utilized. Regardless of the specifics, creating multiple examples will assist you in thoroughly learning a topic and therefore creating a feeling of comfort about your knowledge of the subject.

from worry about doing it and allow you to use this skill to your advantage in your classes as well as in the professional environment.

Most of the fear of speaking in public arises from our fear of appearing the fool. Many students will not ask questions during a lecture specifically because they believe themselves incapable of speaking clearly and identifying exactly the information they need. We have all heard the saying, "There is no stupid question"; we must believe it. You must develop the confidence to speak up when you have a question; consider the potential consequences to your clients should you fail to clarify a medical order or question a procedure that is unclear.

The following strategies may help when you want to ask a question:

- *Understand why you are asking the question.* Instead of saying, "I don't understand," say, "I was with you on the physiology of the kidney until you traveled into the Bowman's capsule. Can you connect this particular part of the kidney with osmosis for me?" This puts you and the speaker in a positive light; you have not attacked the speaker's explanation, and you acknowledge your skill in listening. You are communicating what you need and asking the speaker to help by connecting the two concepts for you.
- *Know when to ask the question.* Writing down those topics on which you need further information may help you decide the correct time to ask a question. If the instructor begins by saying, "Today we will be speaking about pharmacokinetics," and you do not understand the word, stopping her before she has a chance to define the word may not be the most effective strategy. If instead you write down, "What does pharmacokinetics mean?" and listen for the meaning of that word in the context of the lecture, you will most likely hear clues as to the word's meaning. The instructor will use other words, such as *absorption, distribution, metabolism,* and *excretion* to describe what happens to a drug as it goes through the body. When an appropriate time in the presentation comes, review those things that have been said and clarify: "So, Prof. Z., am I correct when I say that pharmacokinetics has to do with the movement of drugs through all the systems of the body?" You will get your answer and your instructor will know from your question that you have been listening.

You must speak clearly and articulate those things you need daily as you attend classes; listen to your instructors; listen to your clients; and transmit information to instructors, colleagues, support staff, doctors, and allied health care team members. Practice both the skills of listening and speaking equally and keep asking questions.

DEVELOP YOUR LEARNING STYLE

The term **learning style** refers to the ways you best receive, process, and assimilate information (knowledge) about a particular subject. In your life as a student, you have probably had both of the following experiences.

You attend class with Professor A for Course 100. The professor arranges the room casually in small groupings and breaks up class time to alternate short lectures with small group work. There is time for a hands-on demonstration of the principle along with actual work-related items used as examples. Professor A allows for student–teacher interchange of ideas and gives credence to experiences of the students during the class discussions. You leave the class exhilarated and with ideas, aware that this content connects with your desired outcome. You plan a review of the notes with a fellow student you met in your class group. You continue to prepare throughout the course and prior to the final, on which you get a B.

The next day you attend Course 200 with Professor B. The room is arranged in rows. Professor B puts up the class outline on the overhead, lectures for 40 minutes, then allows 10 minutes at the end for questions. If you hand him a written question, he will answer it during the next class. You dread his boring presentation and wish that Professor B was more like Professor A. You really do not know anyone in the class with whom to study, you cannot understand the text, and your grades are in the low C to D range. You know you need this class for your major. You try to do your part, but you just can't "get into it."

Think about Professor A, who presents information in a variety of methods—short lecture, small group, hands-on demonstration. As a student, you can grasp the information from whichever method appeals to you. You come away feeling connected to the subject and your classmates and want to continue

PROFESSIONAL TIP

Learning Disabilities

According to the National Center for Learning Disabilities, Inc. (NCLD, 1999), 15% to 20% of the population have some form of learning disability. **Learning disability** is a generic term that refers to a heterogeneous group of disorders manifested as significant difficulties in the acquisition and use of listening, speaking, reading, writing, reasoning, or mathematical abilities.

If you think that having a learning disability will prohibit your success, you are incorrect; you must, however, understand your different abilities. You must know those types of accommodations that will enhance your learning capabilities, and you must be comfortable asking for those things that you need. Accommodations in postsecondary programs are mandated by the federal government; however, the onus to disclose, provide documentation, and request accommodations is on the student. Accommodations are determined on a case-by-case basis. Reasonable accommodations in the classroom may be as simple as having the instructor wear a microphone, being able to use a tape recorder or note taker, or requesting textbook tapes. In the clinical area, all reasonable accommodations are made within the confines of client safety and essential skills needed to participate in a program of study for nursing. A quiet work area and ear protectors may provide quiet for students who are hypersensitive to background noise. Using a computer for writing assignments, note taking in class, and studying may assist students who have difficulty writing. Getting a tutor skilled at working with students with learning disabilities may be another intervention to consider.

Whatever you suspect your needs to be, getting professional testing to ascertain whether you have a disability and to determine any specific accommodations you will need is crucial. Seek the assistance of your instructors, student service personnel, learning center personnel, or call the special education coordinator at the nearest high school. These resources will help you locate an accredited testing agency to provide you with further resources and documentation.

learning about the subject. You are rewarded for your efforts through the academic grade system.

Now consider Professor B, who knows just as much about the subject as does Professor A, but who presents it using only one method—lecture. Lecture is not your preferred learning style, and your ability to clarify your understanding through questions is limited by the class format. Your outcomes on tests are less rewarding, and you begin to avoid putting time into studying the subject all together. You end up thinking that you really do not do well in that subject and consider changing your major.

The difference in the outcomes of the two examples lies in the perceived role of the learner. In these examples, the student relied heavily on the *teacher's* ability to present material in the student's preferred learning style. Remember that *you* are in charge of your learning. Teacher presentations vary in ways that may not appeal to your primary learning style, but you can still learn the information. You must take charge of developing your abilities, increasing your awareness of your preferred learning styles, and implementing some simple strategies to enhance those styles. When you identify the ways that you think and learn most efficiently (learning style), you are using critical thinking (Alfaro-LeFevre, 1999). Every person has a preferred learning style. However, the most successful individuals learn to use all three styles of learning: visual, auditory, and kinesthetic (Chaffee, 1999).

Classification of Learning Styles

Learning styles are cognitive (mental) functions. They refer to the ways you perceive, remember, think, and solve problems: Their focus is *how* you learn as opposed to *what* you learn. Your preference for one style over another can be argued to be both genetic and developmental. Regardless, your awareness of the ways you best learn will affect your learning outcomes.

Learning styles are classified in many different ways. One classification method focuses on the route by which students best perceive and remember information: visual, auditory, or kinesthetic. These divisions are not mutually exclusive; we possess all three, and we use all of them to garner our information. Visual learners make up approximately 65% of the population, auditory learners approximately 30%, and kinesthetic learners approximately 5% (Mind Tools, 1998). To do a quick self-assessment, read the descriptions of the different styles in Figure 2-5

☐ **Visual** learners think in pictures. It does not matter whether they are hearing the information, reading the information, or feeling the information. They take in the information through the senses and store it as visual images. When visual learners want to recall information, they "play the movie" in their brain. Visual learners also relate best to information they have seen written down in texts, in their own notes, in diagrams, and in pictures. A statement such as "I see," or "I get the picture" reflects the style of the visual learner.

☐ **Auditory** learners learn best by hearing and listening. They do not make mental pictures but filter information through listening and repeating skills. They relate best to the spoken word. They may not take notes in class, but rather may ask to tape the lecture. These learners prefer classroom discussion and oral presentations over writing assignments. Speech patterns represent exactly how the auditory learner thinks, "I hear you," "That clicks," "That sounds right," "That rings a bell."

☐ **Kinesthetic** learners learn by touch, movement, imitation, and practice. These learners will process and remember information well if they can touch or feel that which they are studying. These students are easily distracted during lectures, do not think in pictures, and can appear slow in understanding didactic material as it is being presented. They may have to go away and process (manipulate) material by rewriting the notes in a condensed format. These learners like to speak about learning in terms of their feelings, saying things like, "I feel" or "I'd like to get a better handle on this information."

Figure 2-5 Division of Learning Styles (*Adapted from Center for New Discoveries in Learning, Personal Learning Style Inventory, 1998*)

and note the one(s) that come closest to describing the way you prefer to receive information.

You may have selected two or three styles from Figure 2-5, because we sometimes use one style over another in certain learning situations. If all of the noted styles were "close," you may want to rank them to gain a better understanding of your overall learning style. All of us have the capacity to learn in all three modes. You naturally gravitate to one over the others based on which style has led to your greatest learning successes.

Another way to classify learning styles is according to brain-hemisphere dominance. The left hemisphere of the brain is associated with analytical activities, such as logic, structure, speech, reasoning, numbers, verbal expression, verification of data, and analysis of parts of the whole. The right side is associated with creativity and synthesizing parts to form a whole idea. The right side is also considered the more emotional side and links to insight, intuition, daydreams, visualization, music, rhythm, and color visualization.

We need both sides of the brain to function and learn. Numerous studies demonstrated that individuals with left-brain dominance are primarily auditory learners and those with right brain dominance are primarily visual. Additional studies show that right-brain–dominant learners process, recall, and retain more from information presented in computer-assisted instructional programs, whereas left-brain–dominant learners derive more success from a lecture format. To overlook or use one style to the exclusion of the other is using only part of your overall potential learning ability.

Strategies for Learning

By determining your preferred learning style you will be able to adopt strategies to enhance that style when you study. You want to effectively move the required information into long-term memory and increase your knowledge level from memorization to comprehension and, finally, to application. To accomplish this you must know which strategies work with which learning styles. Refer to Table 2-5 and note all of the strategies listed that you consistently use in your study routine. Start with the style you previously ascertained to be your preferred learning style.

Are there strategies listed under your preferred style that you currently do not use? To enhance your acquisition of material, begin to incorporate these into your study plan. Are these strate-

Table 2-5 SAMPLE LEARNING STRATEGIES		
VISUAL LEARNER	**AUDITORY LEARNER**	**KINESTHETIC LEARNER**
Takes notes in class	Reads aloud	Takes notes and rewrites them to condense
Writes notes in margin of book	Reads into a tape recorder and plays it back to self	Expresses self with hands, even while reading
Looks for reference books with pictures, graphs, and charts	Discusses ideas about class content with others	Handles visual aids during class
Draws own illustrations	Requests explanations of illustrations	Requests to do a demonstration

gies listed under any of the other styles that you could use when the material you are learning is especially difficult for you?

One way to incorporate more than one learning style into your study program is to employ a CAI program. Many texts now come with an accompanying disk designed to enhance learning style. Such disks may contain the total text along with testing materials, exercises that accompany the text, and/or resource material for the text. For example, several medical terminology packages come as program-instruction texts with disks and provide audio pronunciation in the computer programs. The student can read the text, manipulate the information on the computer, and hear the correct pronunciation.

To begin to incorporate new learning styles related to the way you receive and recall information, review the list in Table 2-6 and think about ways to add the study strategies to your study plan. You will notice that the three basic learning styles (visual, auditory, and kinesthetic) are expanded on in this list.

When faced with a particularly difficult passage or concept, incorporate more that one style and one strategy to process the information. The more action you put into your learning methods, the more effective your time and outcomes will be.

DEVELOP A TIME-MANAGEMENT PLAN

Somewhere in your decision-making process to go to school, you decided you would have the time to do so. You now must make that a reality by actively engaging in a time-management plan. **Time management** is a system to help meet goals through problem solving. Practicing time-management strategies will not eliminate the need to perform tasks you do not like, but it will make doing so more manageable. Active application of time-management strategies will make a difference in what you can accomplish in the time you have.

Strategies for time management include the following:

- Analyzing your time commitments
- Knowing yourself
- Clarifying your goals
- Setting priorities and identifying one or two valued goals to achieve
- Disciplining yourself to adhere to the plan through changes and until the goal is reached

Table 2-6 ADDITIONAL LEARNING STYLES AND STRATEGIES

STYLE	STUDY TECHNIQUES
Linguistic (word smart: uses words as cues, likes poems)	Speaks out loud, uses audiotapes of text information, uses workbooks, makes up **mnemonics** (words or phrases used to aid memory)
Logical/math (number smart: looks for patterns, enjoys science)	Needs to have a connection for information; uses charts, diagrams, note taking; may use mapping rather than straight words to see connections
Spatial (picture smart: visualizes, good at puzzles)	Draws diagrams; uses flash cards; chooses books with pictures, charts, and diagrams rather than total text, workbooks with pictures; uses highlighters in multiple colors to indicate special things and help information take hold in mind
Body/kinesthetic (body smart: rides a bike, walks, moves, loves the outdoors)	Tapes lectures, walks and listens, watches a video while on the treadmill, goes to a unit to "see" the information, goes to the library to get information, drives and listens to taped lectures or notes (allotted time takes on importance)
Music (music smart: listens to/ loves music, plays an instrument)	Makes up songs and rhymes, uses audiotapes of information or makes up own, listens to music while studying
Interpersonal (people smart: talks things through, likes to chat over coffee)	"Teaches" the material to somebody, studies in a group, runs material by mentor or coworkers
Intrapersonal (self smart: uses quiet time to process, a hobby person)	Uses examples from own experience to apply information, may process material from audiotape while doing a hobby

Adapted from Learning Out of the Box, "Tuning in to Your Unique Cluster of Intelligences," *by K. H. Matthews, 1997, Fall, 22–27 The* Next Step Magazine.

Analyze Time Commitments

To analyze your time commitments, start by listing them. You should provide yourself with both a big-picture plan and a daily plan. Creating a year-at-a-glance calendar that lists all of your important time commitments can provide a quick illustration of the way the months ahead will be used. Start by putting in your graduation date in red capital letters. This will give you an instant visual reminder of your current goal. Next, using a pencil, insert all important dates including holidays, birthdays, work, and organizational obligations. Remember to also include activities for those in your household that will require your participation, such as carpooling, special school programs, after-school activities, and child care. Use your academic program calendar as the source for the dates classes, as well as vacations, begin and end, financial aid forms and tuition payments are due, and the like. Use your individual class schedules as the sources for dates of exams, special review or clinical days, field trips, or any other time commitments that you must meet in order to complete the courses. This exercise will give you a big-picture view of your time commitments and will also point out any conflicts.

Conflicts are not impossible obstacles. Knowing about them in advance will allow you to take steps now to prioritize and reschedule. When prioritizing, think about delegating some tasks to other people. Do not always solve a conflict by removing those tasks you enjoy or that will renew you. Taking care of yourself during this time will be very important. Never give up the time you need to refresh and renew, even if it is just a hot bath, a brisk 15-minute walk, or a dinner out with family and friends. Place yourself near the top of the priority list to complete your goal.

Each learner's big-picture map will differ. The struggle is to mesh your map with your other relationships and keep yourself toward the top of the list. One strategy is to prominently display your big-picture calendar in an area where all of the members of your household can see it—including and especially you. Everyone will then have the opportunity to see that they are on the list and that they contribute to helping you reach your goal.

The next step is daily planning. Using a week-at-a-glance planner helps illustrate more concrete expectations of those things you plan to do and the amount of time you actually have (Figure 2-6). You should include time to sleep, eat, drive, work, attend class, and study.

	Monday	Tuesday	Wednesday	Thursday	Friday	Saturday	Sunday
7 AM	Work	Carpool	Carpool	Carpool	Clinical	House Chores	
9 AM	Work	Class	Class	Class		House	Sunday school
11 AM	Work	Class	Class	Class		Chores	Church
1 PM	Work	Class	Class	Class			
3 PM	Work				Work	Work	
5 PM	Carpool Dinner				Work	Work	
7 PM					Work	Work	

Figure 2-6 Week-at-a-glance Calendar

PROFESSIONAL TIP

Time Wasters

Are you a time waster? We all sometimes behave in ways that sabotage the best of plans. Following are some examples of time wasters along with some strategies for helping you reclaim those wasted hours.

1. *Clutter:* Wisdom holds that you can save 1 hour each day by just clearing your work area of clutter and keeping it clean. This time can be put to good use in the form of study. Organize your study area so that when you arrive it is ready for work, and take a few minutes at the end of your session to prepare your area for the next session.

2. *Interruptions:* Intrusions into your study or work hours (from either people or things) can be real time wasters. Try the following:

   • Learn to say, "no." You do not have to agree to every request. Learn to pick your involvements carefully and according to those which are most important to you reaching your goals.
   • Put your answering machine on, and turn the phone's ringer off. Delegate a time to listen and respond to messages after studying.
   • Open your mail over the garbage can. Respond, delegate, or throw it out.

Professional Tip *continued*

- Organize your papers. For instance, have a folder for each child's paper/notes. Keep your class notebooks, your calendar, and phone lists in one three-ring binder, so you have all your essentials together.

3. *Procrastination:* This refers to intentionally putting off or delaying something that should be done. **Procrastination** is a time waster because it does not afford effective use of time. Time management is not necessarily finishing everything at one sitting, but, rather, scheduling time to return to the task until you complete it; whereas procrastination is intentionally delaying the task without good cause or a plan to complete it in a time-efficient manner. Breaking the task down into manageable segments and rewards will encourage you to return to it again and again until it is complete.

4. *Perfectionism:* Very often we do not stick to a plan because it does not give us results immediately or does not give the results we expected. Perfectionism affects your time-management plan by prohibiting you from accepting anything less than perfection; it also damages your positive attitude of yourself by setting unrealistic expectations. Focus on your positive accomplishments, look for ways to improve, accept your failures, and build on your experiences.

You may find that you must rearrange your schedule. This does not mean continuing to do all of the things you have listed but just on different days; rather, it means choosing two valued goals on which to work. *One must be to be a learner. The other will be unique to you.* This does not mean that you replace all other goals with these two valued goals. Rather, it means that these goals must take precedence when choosing ways to use your time. If you choose child care and learner as your most valued goals, you could refine them even further to complement each other. For example, you may opt to keep driving the carpool, but negotiate to drive every morning, because doing so will afford you 2 hours to study prior to class. You may then have to make child care arrangements for after school, which might mean asking your neighbor or contracting with an after-school program.

You may also have to set aside 1 hour each evening to get everything laid out for the next day, a task you might ask someone else in the household to do each night so that you can gain an extra hour of study time. That extra hour, in turn, might mean that you dedicate Saturdays for nothing but family commitments. Regardless of the way you choose to solve such problems, the solutions must be designed to help you reach your goals.

Know Yourself

To develop your system you must know yourself. You must be honest with yourself about your work habits and preferences. Consider the time of day when you are at your intellectual best. Is it early in the morning, or do you come alive at 10 P.M.? You must be able to focus and concentrate when you are studying. Deciding you are going to carpool in the morning to get to school early to study will not be effective if you cannot concentrate until after noon. If this is the case, it would be better to do the more mechanical and less intellectually demanding tasks, such as the shopping or laundry, in the 2 hours before class. Are you a person who is more left-brain oriented (logical, orderly, structured, and plays by the rules)? Then writing out lists of tasks and crossing them off may be your time-management strategy to stay on track. Perhaps you are a more right-brain personality (creative, resists rules, has own sense of time)? Scheduling your task within a specific time frame that has a time-sensitive goal/reward at the end may assist you to use your available time more effectively.

Clarify the Goal

Without setting goals, we cannot know whether we are making any progress. Goals are like grocery lists. Think about when you go to the store without a list. You may purchase many items, but when you get home you often discover that you did not get all the things you needed. If you make a list the next time you go to the store, however, you will likely get all the items you want.

Just like the grocery list, goals must be written down. They must be based on reality and broken down into manageable parts. Say your goal is to provide study time each week that will allow you to be successful in each unit exam of your program. This time will comprise the time you need to prepare and review material, prepare for clinical assignments, view information in the library, and practice new skills in the lab. As a rule, you will need 1 to 2 hours of study time for each hour you spend in class. If you are in class 12 hours per week, you will thus need to find 24 more hours to study; and if you are in clinical 6 hours 3 days per week for a total of 18 hours, you will need to fit in 36 hours of study. As a rough estimate, this would mean 12 class hours plus 24 study hours plus 18 clinical hours plus 36 preparation hours for a total of 90 hours per week (30 class hours plus 60 study hours) for the ideal study week and 30 hours (class attendance only) for a week without any study. So now you know what amount of time you are aiming for. You can now take this goal of 60 study hours per week and compare it to your written schedule and calendar to determine how to best arrange the demands on your time in order to meet your goals.

Set Priorities

Another part of setting goals is prioritizing tasks into general categories. Look at your daily calendar and list the general categories. Some examples might be as follows:

- Work
- Study
- Personal (eating, sleeping)
- Household chores (shopping, budget)
- Transportation (self, others)
- Supervising children
- Decision making (planning, outside organizational responsibility, time for self, time for spouse, friends, and children)

Next, rank these general categories in order of priority, keeping in mind that not everything is a primary priority. If you uncover conflicts, try to further clarify which items take top priority.

Another way to prioritize is to group tasks according to the time frame in which you wish them to be accomplished. To do this, divide a sheet of paper into three parts. Label the first part column A, the second, column B, and the third, column C. Under column A, write "I must work on these tasks now." This list includes your priority tasks that need immediate attention. Under column B, write "I can do these after A is done." Under column C, write "I can delay, eliminate, or delegate these until after B is done" (Figure 2-7).

If you placed your entire list under column A, go back to your original two goals—one of which includes your new role as learner—and rethink your list. You must prioritize your activities

A	B	C
I must work on these tasks now	I can do these after A is done	I can delay, eliminate, or delegate these until after B is done
school/study	*supervise children*	*organization*
child care		*shopping*
self-care		
work		

Figure 2-7 Prioritizing Tasks

in order to reach your goal. *You cannot be all things at all times to all people.* You also must know how to work smarter, not longer or harder, to remain focused on the priority task.

Discipline Yourself

The hardest strategy to commit to may be the last one. The idea that you must actively engage in using the plan sounds simple. In practice, the plan will not always work. When this happens, you may be tempted to abandon the plan instead of changing it. If the plan is not working, you must ascertain the reasons. Maybe you lack resources, have not scheduled enough time, or need to revisit and reevaluate your goal. Build time to plan into your weekly schedule. If you really want to use a time-management system, your ability to go back to the plan and revise it will be very important.

DEVELOP A STUDY STRATEGY

Developing a study plan involves more than just buying a textbook and reading it. Several strategies that will assist you to study more efficiently and effectively follow.

Appropriate Learning Attitude

Many students allow themselves to have a negative or self-critical attitude, as expressed by these statements: "This is too much to learn." "I'll never be able to learn this." "I've never been a good student." These attitudes undermine a student's learning efforts.

To develop a positive, realistic attitude toward learning, students should seriously appraise their abilities and commitment to learning. Students who adopt an attitude that they *will* be successful will work to make this prediction come true.

Set Up the Environment

Where and when you study are as important as how. The fact that you assign a specific behavior to your study space will set you up for success. The space should fit your style. Do you like everything organized in neat spaces, or do you just need it near you? What type of lighting, seating, or noise level will assist or detract from your concentration? Consider your preferred learning style when setting up your study space (Figure 2-8). If you are a kinesthetic learner, you may want to put motion into your space by, for instance, using a treadmill in your study plan. You may want to spend a percentage of your study time sitting to read and take notes and then switch to walking or running on the treadmill to recite and reflect on the material. You will be increasing comprehension and making connections, all while walking 2 miles! Regardless of the way you arrange your space, take into consideration the type of learner you are and your biological and personality preferences.

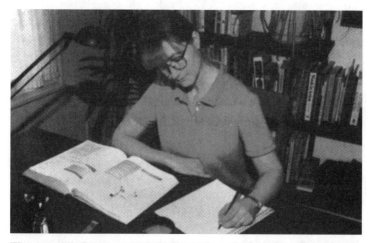

Figure 2-8 Create a study space that reflects your learning style. Ensure that all the resources you need to study are close at hand. (*Photo courtesy of Tom Stock*)

Gather Your Resources

Your resources should all be easily accessible from your study space. In some homes, the kitchen table serves as the study space. If your study space serves more than one function, as would the kitchen table, consider keeping your study resources in a milk crate or box so they are portable yet readily at hand when needed.

Gathering your resources is your start to building a library of textbooks, which will serve you throughout your program. These resources become a reference library for you when you study. Some general resources to keep on hand include the following:

- A recent edition of an unabridged dictionary
- A medical dictionary
- An anatomy and physiology text

Additional resources you will need as you progress through your program may include texts on pharmacology, nutrition, and the nursing process. Depending on your personal knowledge base, you may need further resources in the foundation sciences—biology, psychology, and sociology. These areas serve as the knowledge base for your future profession.

Keeping your learning style in mind, consider purchasing accompanying workbooks or other study aids that come with the text and research CAI or videotapes available in your nursing program library. Using varied and multiple resources enhances your knowledge base and will increase your comprehension of the content. You must go beyond memorization, beyond amassing facts, to comprehension of this knowledge base in order to answer the questions on the exams. Keep in mind that you are studying for the program examination, the National Council Licensure Examination (NCLEX-PN), and, ultimately, to apply your knowledge base to provide safe, effective care to your clients.

Remember to use journals as resources. The articles and related client situations can assist you in understanding the application of content to the clinical area. Your ultimate goal is to apply your content information to client care. Consider getting a subscription to your nursing journal, *The Journal of Practical Nursing*. Nursing organizations such as the National Federation of Licensed Practical Nursing are also valuable resources, and many have web sites, which you can visit.

Whatever resources you ultimately choose, gathering them and having your resources readily at hand are simple strategies that will make the time you have allotted for study more efficient and effective.

Minimize Interruptions

Interruptions to your study time decrease the actual time you can focus on the material and affect your concentration. Interruptions may also become your procrastination "triggers." If you allow your study time to be constantly interrupted, you will soon be doing something other than studying. At the very least, these interruptions minimize your efficient use of time. When you plan your time to study, do not set yourself up for interruptions. Look realistically at your time schedule and do not schedule your study time around the household's "naturally" busy times of the day—typically mornings, mealtimes, early evenings, and bedtimes.

This is where you put the strategies listed in the section on time management to work. If you have set aside a time and a space for study, make it known that you are not to be interrupted unless there is an emergency. Hang a sign on the door that reads, "Think, before you knock." Planning on studying in 1 or 1½ hour blocks is also a way to cut down on interruptions. This is a reasonable time period for you to put the world on hold in order to accomplish your task.

Get to Know the Textbook

Your textbook is not intended to be read like the latest mystery novel, from beginning to end in one sitting. It has both directions on the way to use it (introduction, preface) and built-in references (glossary, appendix, summary questions). It is arranged in sections, each dealing with a major topic, and then subdivided into the parts (chapters) that make up the sum of that topic. Getting to know your textbook and its resources and the author's approach to writing may constitute the first part of your study plan. Having this information gives you some insight into the way the material has been grouped and connected.

Another author may have written the book in totally stand-alone chapters and may encourage students to review the table of contents and start anywhere they feel they need to. Self-instruction modules or texts in math often give students instructions to first take all of the posttests in the chapters and as long as a certain score is reached, to go on. This is a means of giving students credit for knowledge already learned and facilitating recall of knowledge in preparation for new learning.

Take a look at various parts of this text. How is the information organized? What built-in references can assist you? Consider the cues given about the way to use this text to help you organize the big picture.

Set Up the Study Plan

Each time you enter your study "space," your study plan should be with you. You should have a plan or a specific goal for that time. Each time you enter the space, bring a positive attitude toward reaching that goal. Your nursing course outline will drive your study plan. You will have a certain amount of material to cover in a specific time span. You first must know those things that are expected of you. Your course outline, curriculum, and instructors will give you this information.

As an example, consider a unit on vital signs, which is assigned to be completed in 1 week. The components of the unit include understanding the theory base about vital signs as well as learning the psychomotor skills involved in actually measuring these indicators. You are expected to acquire the knowledge by reading the chapter in the text, attending the lecture and demonstration, and practicing in the lab. You will be tested on your ability to apply your knowledge through a pencil-and-paper test and a redemonstration of your psychomotor skills. Now that you know the information you must cover, the sources of the information, and the way you will be tested, you can map out a study plan. Consider the following steps:

1. *Preview the material to be studied.* Your assigned reading from the text on the content of the unit may be contained in one chapter or may span several chapters. Always preview the assigned chapter(s). Often, the student reads only the pages assigned, thinking that this is the most efficient way to study. By not spending the 5 or 10 minutes to preview the entire chapter, the connections between the content may be lost. Previewing can be done very quickly by scanning the chapter headings, art, and tables.

2. *Consider the chapter heading.* The material about vital signs may be contained in a chapter labeled "Baseline Assessment" or "Measurement of Baseline Values" or "Physiologic Functions of the Body." All of these give you a cue as to what you are about to study.

3. *Read the objectives for the chapter.* The objectives list those things you should be able to do when you are finished learning the content of the chapter.

4. *Scan the vocabulary section and the end-of-chapter summary and questions.* Read the key terms and the summary and questions at the chapter's end. Doing so gives you an overview of the scope of the reading you will need to do and should take no more than 5 to 10 minutes.

5. *Set up your questions.* Beginning at the chapter objectives, write down those things you already know, questions about those things you must learn for each objective, and some additional resources that you think you should check. For example, in a chapter about vital signs, the initial page may look like the one in Figure 2-9. Jot down your current knowledge, your questions. The resources note relates to the reasons you are trying to learn this material. Connecting the material to your role in the profession is most important. You are now ready to read the chapter critically for the answers to your questions. You may uncover more and have more questions at the end; but you have a plan and can move on to the next step.

6. *Read and take notes.* Answer your questions and check your vocabulary knowledge as you read.

7. *Reread when necessary.* Remember your basic skills and concentration.

8. *Reflect on the connections you can make between the material and client care.* Identify the reasons the information is important and the way you will use it.

9. *Recite or create your individual style cues.* This is where you will put your individual unique learning styles to work. Make up songs. Create mnemonics. Design flash cards for items that must be memorized. Try to create a logical connection when recalling information.

10. *Review or summarize the information.* Answer the objectives. Use your own words to answer your initial questions. Do you have more questions? Must you consult a second resource to answer them?

11. *End the session with a critical thinking question.* What would the client look like if his temperature were 103°F? What other body systems would be affected? What nursing measures might I use to support the client with this level temperature (e.g., monitor the client's fluid intake and output because the body would be losing fluid as a result

The Measurement of Vital Signs

At the completion of this chapter, you should be able to:

1. Describe the physiologic mechanisms controlling temperature, pulse, respiration, and blood pressure.

   Temp = ?, Pulse = heart, Respiration = lungs,
   Blood pressure = arteries need to find out about temp.

2. Identify the normal range for vital sign measurements.

   For adults? Children?

3. Select the appropriate equipment used to take vital signs.

   Thermometer, stethoscope, blood pressure cuff

4. Demonstrate the correct psychomotor technique used in measuring vital signs.

   I do this in the lab/get procedure from book or instructor?
   Ask in class.

5. Document the normal findings of the measurement of blood pressure.

   Temp = 98.6, p = 60-80, bp = 120/80
   I need to know this to be able to tell if the client
   is normal or having trouble.

Figure 2-9 Start with the chapter objectives and devise questions and answers to determine those things that you know and those things that you will need to give more attention.

of the thermoregulation [sweating and evaporation that would reduce the temperature]), and why? Write these down in your notes. You will soon have a collection of "client scenarios" that you will be able to build on as you increase your knowledge base.

The preceding steps require skill in five areas: reading, rereading, reflecting, reciting, and review. With each step, you are engaging in the process of encoding the material. **Encoding** is thought of as actually laying down tracks in the areas of your brain. Each time you read, reread, reflect, recite, and review, you increase the depth of the tract, and your ability to recall and utilize the information increases. You move the information from short-term to long-term memory, and you increase your level of knowledge. The more senses and action you put into your study plan, the more you are able to utilize the information.

You move your level of knowledge from the memorization of a group of facts to the comprehension of the facts in a logical, organized fashion that allows you to relate the information to clients to whom you will provide care. Each time you sit down to study, this should be your goal. You can preview, question, and quickly outline the major points in the chapters prior to class. Listen to the lecture and take notes. Approach new material with the read, reread, reflect, recite, and review steps before moving on to the next topic.

Note Taking

Note taking is an action that connects you to the content of written material or a lecture presentation and will assist you in identifying the main ideas and their connection to the overall topic.

Keep materials for each of your classes or topics in a separate three-ring binder. Take notes on loose-leaf paper and write on one side only, as this allows you to arrange your preview notes and lecture notes chronologically. You can also insert handouts from the class in the appropriate order as you receive them. Using this method, you can also review notes against additional information you have from other resources to assist you when it is time to review for the examinations.

When you are taking notes from the text, read with a pencil in your hand to put yourself in the action mode. You will thus be ready to receive and process information. You may also take notes from text readings on your computer, which facilitates editing and rearranging material.

Prior to class, preview your chapter material and divide your paper, leaving a 3-inch border on the left side. From the assigned reading, identify the main topic to be covered, list the main section and the subheadings, and summarize the information in the left column. Then write your questions in this column. This prepares you for more active participation in the lecture; use the right column to take notes from the lecture.

Regardless of the way you choose to take notes, note taking while you study sets you up for connecting with the content. It positions you as an active participant in the learning process, and any time you increase your active participation in the learning process, you increase your learning.

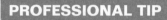

PROFESSIONAL TIP

Mnemonics

Create your own mnemonics to group the steps of a procedure. A mnemonic is simply a method for helping your association and recall; it consists of a memorable word or phrase created from the letters of the list of items you are trying to recall. For example, to remember all of the areas to include when assessing a client to whom a cast has been applied (pulse, circulation, sensation, movement, and temperature), you might make up a silly sentence to help you remember, such as "*P*aul *C*an *S*hine *M*y *T*uba." This type of statement will help you group these facts together (pulse, circulation, sensation, movement, temperature) and assist you in recalling them. You could sing this also. Do whatever you can to be active in moving material from short-term to long-term memory.

When taking notes in class, listen attentively, lean forward, and concentrate on the information the speaker is imparting (Figure 2-10). Take notes on the following:

- The topic, as stated by the speaker; write it on the top of the page
- The main ideas and the details that support the topic
- The most important points, based on the speaker's organization and emphasis
- Other students' questions and the responses from the speaker, which are often the very questions you had

Look for visual and auditory cues from the speaker, for example, if the speaker says, "This is important" or writes steps on the board. Do not form an opinion of what is being said until you have heard the entire lecture. As stated earlier, a good strategy is to write your questions as you think of them. They may be answered by the time the lecture is over.

The purpose of note taking during a lecture is not to create a transcript of the information imparted, but, rather, to record what you understand. The combination of attending lecture, listening, and note taking can provide you with much knowledge that you will not have to learn elsewhere. Previewing the

PROFESSIONAL TIP

Memory and Activity

Remember the following as a guide for a study plan when you want to learn new material:

People Remember	Learner Activity
10% of what they *READ*	Reading
20% of what they *HEAR*	Hearing the words
30% of what they *SEE*	Watching still pictures (charts, diagrams)
50% of what they *SEE and HEAR*	Watching moving pictures (video or a demonstration)
70% of what they *SAY and WRITE*	Giving a presentation/ making up a story (case studies)
90% of what they *SAY AS THEY PERFORM THE EXPERIENCE*	Talking your way through a demonstration Teaching someone else

Adapted from Audiovisual Methods in Teaching *(p. 43), by E. Dale, 1954, New York: Dryden Press.*

material to be covered further contributes to this dynamic. When taking notes, consider the following guidelines to make your note taking efficient and effective:

- Do not take notes with the intent of writing them over. This is a waste of time and, contrary to what you may expect, it does not improve recall. Making a note map of your notes is a more effective recall tool.
- If your handwriting is sloppy, print or use a laptop computer.
- Condense the amount of actual writing you do by using symbols and abbreviations and leaving out everything but necessary words. For instance, instead of writing "If the client's blood pressure reading is greater than 140 systolic and 90 diastolic, . . . " write "If BP > 140/90 . . . "
- Write definitions and mathematical formulas exactly as you heard them in lecture.

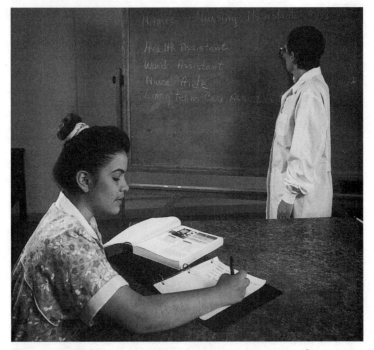

Figure 2-10 Note taking is an important component of increasing your comprehension of the material.

- In mathematics and science lab courses, write the process step by step exactly as explained. Indicate which formulas are used with which problems, for example

    "Use ratio/proportion for word problems"

- Pick an abbreviation system and stick to it.
- Review the notes as soon as possible after class. Many studies have demonstrated that even a brief review of notes after class increases retention of the material by 50%.

Prepare for Exams

The final plus of having a study plan is the ability to review for exams. Reviewing for exams is not studying all of the material over from the beginning. You will already have learned the subject matter you are going to cover on the exam; now, you are reviewing and recalling it through a series of exercises designed to increase your comprehension and facilitate application. Most nursing examinations are written at the comprehen-

PROFESSIONAL TIP

Attending Lectures
In general, the best strategies for getting the most from lectures are to:

- Get to class on time.
- Get a front row seat.
- Listen attentively with a pencil in your hand and take notes.

sion or recall level. The NCLEX-PN is written at the application level. On this exam you will not see many questions about naming where the pulse points are (comprehension, recall), for instance. You will instead find questions about which of the pulse points of the body are most appropriate for assessing an infant (application). Making decisions about which fact or groups of principles you have learned will be the basis for most nursing examination questions.

Depending on the curriculum, you may have examinations every week or every month, a weekly quiz, a midterm, and a final. Regardless, you will know the schedule, and you must set aside review time for preparation. If you are to have weekly quizzes, you must build a time for review into your daily study plan. One way to do so is to set aside the last 30 minutes of each study session for review. Take each objective of your course outline and, without looking at your notes or text, turn them into questions and then answer them. If you are weak in one area, refer to your notes and devise a technique for recall, such as the use of flash cards, rhythms, mnemonics, pictures, or graphic drawings. Work through each of the objectives for the content that will be covered.

If your examinations are by unit, you must divide the material up over the time you will need to cover it, leaving at least 2 days for review and recall prior to the examination. Each of these review sessions will also serve as preparation for both your final examination and the NCLEX-PN. As you are successful in each of your examinations and continue to see further connections in your clinical application, your depth as well as breadth of content mastery will increase.

PRACTICE THINKING CRITICALLY

Most of this chapter thus far has been devoted to presenting strategies for the effective and efficient acquisition of knowledge. Your ultimate goal is to be able to use this knowledge to provide safe client care. To do so, you must go beyond the initial stage of simply acquiring information. In delivering nursing care, facts alone do not constitute a sufficient knowledge base for making sound decisions about client care. You must internalize these facts and be able to manipulate them when presented with new situations.

Your progress in this cognitive arena will be evaluated by testing. Practicing thinking critically will enhance your ability to increase your level of knowledge

You must think about *how* you think. Thinking is a process: It is the way you move information from one point to another to get something accomplished. Have you ever been asked, "How did you arrive at that conclusion?" Your explanation was an example of your thinking process. This process of examining how we think is called **metacognition** (from *meta,* meaning "among" plus *cognition,* meaning "the process of knowing").

Consider all the problem solving you have done in your life. How did you arrive at your decisions? Why did you make the choices you did? Given more information, would you have made different decisions? Have you made decisions you regretted?

To make sound decisions, you must consider the knowledge you have and choose that which is relevant given the unique parameters of the given situation. Each client situation is unique. Your text and instructors present information about nursing practice within what is called *predictable parameters,* but clients are anything but predictable.

In considering which actions you may need to take in a new situation, you must consider past experience and principles of care, postulate possible outcomes from a variety of interventions, and seek additional information from colleagues, clients, and resource materials. This process is called *thinking critically,* and it is what you will be expected to do with the knowledge you are acquiring.

How do you foster this type of thinking and knowledge advancement as you are studying? The following strategies used during your study process will help develop your critical thinking skills.

1. *Recall the facts.* Remind yourself of those things you already know about the targeted topic. (***Example:*** The cardio-

vascular system is made up of the heart, the arteries, and the veins; it carries the blood to the cells.)

2. *Group facts into a pattern and organize the data.* (***Example:*** The heart is the center of this system. The arteries carry blood from the heart to the cells, the veins carry blood from the cells to the heart. The blood's function is to transport nutrients and oxygen to the cells and to take waste and carbon dioxide from the cells.)

3. *Associate this information with an experience or an action.* (***Example:*** The cardiovascular system is like a plumbing system, with the heart as the main pumping station, the arteries as the carriers of the hot water, and the veins as the carriers of the cold water.)

4. *Practice "what if" scenarios.* Imagine a person in your life and analyze the facts that you have learned in light of this person. Confirm whether the facts are applicable. If not, what was significant in this situation to alter your conclusion? What action might you take? (***Example:*** What happens when the pump doesn't work [as in Uncle Joe's pacemaker]? What causes this? What runs the heart's electrical system? What else can cause the main pump to stop working—no food [nutrients] or no oxygen? Where does the heart get its oxygen? How does this affect Joe's lifestyle? How could I tell whether a person has a pacemaker? What would I do if the pacemaker stopped?)

5. *Discuss these questions with peers and your instructor.* Conferring with others increases your experience and the variety of ways you look at a problem and promotes increased comprehension of the subject.

6. *Postulate new solutions.* Allow yourself to consider all possible solutions without assigning merit. There is no need to label an idea as "good" or "bad" before the idea has even been discussed. Often, such flashes of insight come when we are daydreaming, on the verge of sleep, or as we awaken. Our mind is free to roam and process during these times.

The last strategy will involve taking some risk, but students who take that risk quickly develop a thick skin and are the most likely to contribute innovatively to clinical practice as a result of their thinking process. Chapter 1 on critical thinking provides much more information on this particular process, but the subject bears inclusion here. Practice this habit as you study, and never stop asking, "Why?" and "What about this?"

DEVELOP TEST-TAKING SKILLS

Testing is not studying; however, the skills you need for testing are similar to those needed for studying. The task involved in taking a test is not to pass it; to pass the test is the *outcome*. You cannot achieve the outcome if you do not know the task. The task is to read the question, understand what the question is asking, and make a decision about a correct response.

To hone your test-taking behaviors, you must first perform a personal analysis with regard to your attitudes, preparation methods, and behaviors related to a testing situation. Only after you have identified these variables can you initiate strategies to improve your outcomes.

Attitude and Expectations

If you are like most students, you may feel quite anxious about taking a test. You may think of each test as the final chance to show your worth. Or you may consider receiving less than an A on an examination as being the same as failing. Neither of these is a reasonable expectation for testing. Testing is a useful tool for both measuring your level of knowledge and showing what you still need to learn. Have you ever considered that receiving a grade of C on an examination usually indicates that you know 75% of all of the knowledge that was tested? And the knowledge on any given test does not represent all the knowledge you possess. Your attitude toward testing is very important if you are to improve your outcome. Maintaining a reasonable expectation regarding both the purpose of the test as well as the meaning of your grade is often a key factor in improving your test performance.

Preparation

In analyzing your preparation for test taking, you must critically examine your study habits. Review the section in this chapter on study strategies and consider whether you are on task when it comes to your study habits. There may be some areas where you can improve. If you know of an area of weakness, make a conscious effort to develop this part of your preparation. Be reasonable in your expectations and do not expect to see results overnight. Building your study habits takes time and persistence. Persevere and your outcome on tests will improve.

Next, consider the way you review for an examination. Do you cram the night before, or are you consistently planning for questions in your study plan and adding time for review of material prior to the examination? One strategy is to use the technique of note mapping to help you organize the material into manageable parts. Taking each part and developing a more detailed one-page outline that you can take with you to review for 15 to 20 minutes at a time is another method to try. Another suggestion is to change your study place and times. Instead of 1-hour sessions, break your review sessions into 30-minute recall sessions. You must draw an imaginary line between studying and reviewing. Studying is the learning of new knowledge; reviewing comprises recall, organization, and summary of information.

Do not study only just prior to the test. This represents poor technique. What are the odds that prior to the examination you would hit upon just the right information that would be on the test in just the exact form that you would see it on the test? Approaching preparation in this manner serves only to put a few facts into short-term memory. Better to spend the time before the examination relaxing with a good book or good friends or at the spa or gym. You must be confident and rested and come to the testing area with that "good" feeling that results from doing something you like.

Consider the rest you get the night prior to the examination. Physical stamina is needed for concentration. If you cram for a test by "pulling an all-nighter," you are setting yourself up for possible errors on the examination. Be reasonable, revisit your study plan, and get adequate rest.

Next, consider whether you have enough energy to take the test. You can eat what you want, but eat. The cells of the brain require glucose to function; this glucose is supplied in the calories you consume. Try not to increase caffeine intake immediately prior to a test, as doing so may make you jittery.

Finally, ask yourself whether surrounding yourself with positive people helps keep you focused, or whether talking to students prior to a test only makes you more anxious. If the latter is the case, you should arrive with just enough time to walk into the testing room and you should not speak to anyone.

Minimize Anxiety

Anxiety is the physiologic response of the autonomic nervous system to a perceived stressful situation. As the situation becomes more stressful, the body's response increases. This affects the ability to process information and make rational choices. People are often not good at identifying what they are feeling and are often unaware of the degree to which stress affects the ability to take tests.

You must develop a plan to deal with anxiety. Anxiety about our performance is always with us. Past experience with testing often contributes to the development of test anxiety. If our expectation regarding our performance on a test is not mirrored in the grade we receive, our confidence in our ability is shaken,

PROFESSIONAL TIP

The 30-Second Vacation

For those of you who need an "anxiety buster," consider a "30-second vacation." The 30-second vacation is based on a guided imagery technique that is used often in the client care arena. This technique takes practice. Start by doing the following:

Sit in a comfortable spot where you will not be disturbed, close your eyes, and think of an event or a place that evokes a feeling of calmness (not necessarily happiness). This is an event or place that made you feel like everything was right with the world and with you. It can be from any time in your life.

It may take some time to settle on the right event or place. Relax and take a few minutes now and think.

Once you have it, don't tell anyone! This is your secret place, your place of peace, and when you go there, no one can find you.

Once you have selected this event or place, start to give it "life." To do this, you must begin to recall this event or place regularly. Practice doing so at the beginning of your study sessions, when you are stuck in traffic, when you are at the dentist, when you have something difficult to do, at the beginning of your test-taking exercises, or at the beginning of your real tests.

Each time you recall your event or place, give it more "life." Recall the time of day, the setting, the colors of that day. Was it raining, was it sunny, was it snowing? If it was raining, was it a summer rain or an autumn rain? Recall what you were wearing and what colors you had on. Were you alone or with others? Were you eating something? What did the food smell like?

and we approach the whole experience with more and more anxiety.

To deal with anxiety, consciously develop an activity to counter the feeling that anxiety evokes. Some people listen to music, pace, or do deep breathing to combat feelings of stress and anxiety. All of these are good strategies, even if all of them cannot be done *while you are actually taking the test.*

Improve Test-Taking Skills

How do you improve your test-taking skills? You practice, practice, practice and analyze, analyze, analyze. Consider the following:

> *Treat every wrong answer as a treasure. Examine it and discover the secret of why you got it wrong.*

This is the only way to know which errors you are making. From this point forward, always request to review your examinations, and track your incorrect responses using the analysis worksheet presented in Figure 2-11. Initially when you review your tests, do not concern yourself with the content of the questions. Simply write the number of the question in the row that indicates the reason you got that question incorrect. You will also notice that there is a heavy black line before the last row of the worksheet. The first four rows represent what are known as *mechanical errors*; these can be eliminated by developing positive habits and revising current practices. You will notice after 3 or 4 quizzes that a pattern starts to emerge. Imagine that you just took a 100-question test and received a score of 60/100. You then use the worksheet to categorize your incorrect responses.

Of the 40 incorrect answers you provided, you see that 10 of them fell in "did not read carefully," 2 in "did not know the vocabulary," 7 in "inferred additional data," 4 in "identified priorities incorrectly," and 7 in "did not know the material." If you could eliminate the bad habits that resulted in the first 23 errors, this would improve your test score immediately. Your grade would be 83/100. More importantly, tests would truly represent only what you did not know, not areas where bad habits resulted in poor test scores.

After you have identified your error patterns, you can work on developing the counter habits that will eliminate them. Work first on the one that is the most glaring.

Test Question Analysis Worksheet

Reason for Incorrect Response	Test 1 Date	Test 2 Date	Test 3 Date	Test 4 Date	Test 5 Date	Test 6 Date	Test 7 Date	Test 8 Date
Did not read carefully (missed details, missed key words)								
Did not know the vocabulary (medical terminology, English vocabulary)								
Inferred additional data (made assumptions, "read into the question")								
Identified priorities incorrectly (placed events in wrong order)								
Did not know the material								

Figure 2-11 Test Question Analysis Worksheet

Read Carefully

Reading carefully is a test-taking behavior that must be practiced. The section on study strategies noted the value of scanning in looking for important words when you read. When you are reading a test question, however, you must *never* scan. Many students choose incorrect responses because they miss key words, scan the question for familiar terms, infer what the question is, or misinterpret words they read too quickly. Incorrect responses resulting from any of these actions represent poor reading habits rather than a substandard knowledge base. The following exercise will help improve your reading habits.

Exercise for Improving Your Literal Reading Skills

You will need

- A timer (stove/egg).
- An NCLEX-PN review text or any comparable question and answer book. It is important that you have the answers and the rationales for each answer in a review text.
- Two sheets of paper: one to take the test on and one to make your analysis worksheet.
- Pencil or pen.
- Dictionary.

1. Pick a time and a place where there will be no interruptions for 20 minutes. You may neither speak to anyone nor get up to use any other resources. You are taking a test.
2. Randomly pick a page of the review book and choose five questions from that page. It does not matter whether you have studied the content in your program.
3. Set the timer for 5 minutes.
4. Start the test. Read each question out loud.
   a. If you read "over" a word, stop reading, make a mark next to that word, and begin again from the beginning.
   b. If you mispronounce a word, stop reading, make a mark next to that word, and begin again from the beginning.
   c. If you do not know the meaning of a word (English or medical), stop and look it up.
5. At the end of the question, restate what is being asked of you.
6. Read the choices, connect each to the question, and choose the most correct answer.

7. When the timer goes off, score your questions.
8. Analyze why you got questions correct or incorrect.
9. Repeat this exercise with five different questions three or four times a week.

The object of this exercise is not to finish all the questions, nor is it even to get all the answers right. Rather, the object is to consciously practice reading every word literally. Each time you do this exercise, you must treat it as a test—no food, no talking, no music, no interruptions. You must associate this type of reading with taking a test, so that each time you take a test, this literal reading habit is instinctual.

Know the Vocabulary

If vocabulary is your weak area, there is only one thing to do—learn the vocabulary. Look up the word (English and medical) in the appropriate dictionary, write the definition on the back of your analysis sheet, and review the definition during your next study session. Add additional time in your study plan for vocabulary building. Use additional modes of learning such as audio or flashcards to master your vocabulary skills.

Do Not Infer Additional Data

The more experiences you have in life, the easier it is to infer additional data in any given situation. You must realize, however, that for the moment, the only relevant information is the information on the test paper—no more, no less. Based on that information alone and the given choices, you must decide on the correct responses. You base your decision on those things you have learned about the topic, on standards of care, on the nursing process, and on your base of knowledge. If you read into the question, you have in essence rewritten it and may not choose the correct answer. One strategy for overcoming this habit is to recognize whenever you begin to interject information upon getting to the last word in a question. In any such instance, you must stop, take some physical action to call your attention to the fact that you are adding information, and clear your mind—take a breath, clear your throat, wear a rubber band and snap it! Then start over again, concentrating on reading the question literally.

Identify Priorities Correctly

When questions concern priorities, ask yourself which of the given choices would result in serious consequences if not done first. When you are being questioned about procedural tasks, ask which of the given choices must be done before the others.

Know the Material

Not knowing the material represents a lack of knowledge base. Write down the content area of each of the questions you miss, then go back and review the concept or facts in question. If the same content areas are problematic over several tests, seek additional assistance from your instructor. You need clarification regarding your understanding of both the information and the questions.

Behaviors in the Testing Room

Setting yourself up in the testing room for a positive experience can make a difference in your outcome. Be sure to practice the following behaviors:

1. *Get a good seat.* Unless your seat is assigned, sit in an area that is quiet, has good light, and where you can "zone in" on the test and "zone out" the rest of the room. If you are a student who gets anxious when you are the last one left in the room, pick a seat in the front row and farthest from the door and turn your seat slightly toward the wall. You will be less apt to notice as people leave.

2. *Set the mood.* As you wait for the test to be passed out, take your 30-second vacation. Adopt the most positive attitude possible. Identify the task ahead of you. Take a breath and repeat the following:

   "I have prepared. I am able to read the questions, process the information, and, from the choices given, make the best choice and move on."

3. *Read—do not scan.* You must read literally every word in the question. Every word counts!

4. *Read the question to determine the following:*
   - *Who is the question about?* This will affect your chosen answer. If you automatically assume that all of the questions relate to the nurse, you may miss a question that asks you to decide those things the father might say to demonstrate his understanding of the discharge instructions, for example.
   - *What is the question about?* You must determine to which part of the knowledge base the question refers. Is the question about the way to teach a 9-year-old juvenile diabetic

to check his blood glucose? To answer this question, you must consider the learning style of the 9-year-old, his cognitive development and manual dexterity, and any significant others who should be involved in the session. The correct choice must support all of these principles.

- *When is the question about?* The time frame of the question is also significant in terms of the client's continuum of care. Is this the acute session? Is this a client who has had diabetes for 20 years and is now developing pulmonary vascular disease? Is this a new mother with her first child or a new mother with her fifth? Are you in the assessment phase of the nursing process, are you in the planning stage, or are you evaluating the effects of a treatment or a drug?

- *Where is the question about?* The focus of the nurse in the acute care institution is different from that of the nurse in the community clinic. This will affect your choice.

5. *Do not argue with the question.* Whether you agree with the question is irrelevant. The task is to read the question, put your mind to the question, and, given the choices offered, make your choice based on principles and the application of your knowledge base.

6. *Plan your time.* Do not spend an inordinate amount of time on one question. There are some things you will not know, and if you spend so much time on one question, you can sabotage your success on others. You can come back to any question, but you must be able to clear your mind of this question before moving on to tackle another. This is a good place for a 30-second vacation to put you back on task! If you cannot let a question "go," you will be unable to concentrate on the next few questions and, very likely, will get several questions in a row incorrect. It is best to read, choose, and move on.

7. *Do not panic.* When you come to a question that you cannot immediately answer, do not panic. Use your 30-second vacation to counter your anxiety and facilitate your ability to process. Recite again, "I have prepared, I am able to read, process, choose, and move on." Remember, the answer is on the paper.

Test-Taking Strategies

There are some basic test-taking strategies that can be used with various types of test questions. These strategies assist critical thinking when answering test questions. They cannot take the place of studying and preparing for a test. Never change an answer unless you are positive it was marked incorrectly. Look over the entire test and plan the approximate time for each question or section of the test based on the time allowed for the test.

Multiple Choice Test Strategies

- Read all answers before choosing one.
- Give extra consideration to long answers especially if words such as *usually, probably, many*, or *some* are used.
- Be wary of answers using words such as *always, never*, or *everyone*.
- Make an educated guess, do not leave questions unanswered.
- Select one of the middle answers when guessing.

True/False Test Strategies

- *All* parts of the statement must be true to answer true; if not, the answer is false.
- Negative words and double negatives must be read very carefully.
- Be careful of long, complex statements.
- Statements using words such as *usually, probably, many*, or *some* are many times true.
- Statements using words such as *always, never*, or *everyone* are generally false.
- When guessing, select true.

Matching Test Strategies

- Read both lists first.
- Mark the matches you are sure of and cross off with a pencil.
- Then work with the matches you are not sure of.

Short Answer Test Strategies

- Check the point value for each question.
- Look at the amount of space provided for the answer.
- Be concise and specific.

Essay Test Strategies

- Read the question carefully.
- Mark key words in the question.

- Take time to think of ideas to answer the question.
- Organize key points in an outline or mapping format.
- Support the key points with explanations and reasons. Use critical thinking.
- Respond to each part of the question.

SUMMARY

- Developing a positive attitude will enhance your learning experience.
- Strategies for developing a positive attitude include creating a positive self-image, recognizing your abilities, and identifying realistic expectations for meeting those goals.
- Nurses must develop competency in the basic skills of reading, arithmetic and mathematics, writing, listening, and speaking.
- It is important to build your vocabulary and comprehension of medical terminology to better enable you to meet your clients' learning needs.
- Should you suspect that you have a learning disability, it is important to identify the disability so that you can seek the right tools to help compensate for the disability.
- The most common learning styles are visual, auditory, and kinesthetic.
- Identifying your preference for a particular learning style will help you identify the strategies you need to be a successful student.
- Organizing your study space and decreasing interruptions will increase your efficiency and facilitate your sticking to your study plan.
- Several methods can be used to take notes. Note taking in lectures and from your text is a strategy to help you retain the information presented.
- Critical thinking is the ability to apply your knowledge base.
- Developing a strategy to minimize anxiety when taking tests will improve your performance.
- To successfully complete a test, read each question thoroughly, do not infer additional information, and identify priorities.

Review Questions

1. Ninety percent of your program is based on which basic skill?
   a. listening
   b. writing
   c. reading
   d. mathematics

2. What is a sign of true comprehension of material?
   a. the ability to repeat a paragraph word for word
   b. memorization of the material
   c. the ability to recite the material
   d. the ability to summarize the material using your own words

3. If you suspect you have a learning disability, it is important that you:
   a. ignore it; you will be able to work around it on your own.
   b. be tested to determine the assistance you will need to compensate for the disability.
   c. keep it to yourself; you will not be able to pass the program if you tell anyone about it.
   d. use it as an excuse to put less work into the program.

4. A kinesthetic learner:
   a. learns by using the senses and visual images.
   b. learns by movement and imitation.
   c. learns by hearing and listening.
   d. learns by example.

5. The best way to study is to:
   a. read only the assigned material.
   b. take notes in the lecture only.
   c. read, reread, reflect, recite, and review.
   d. read and attend lectures.

6. What is the best way to deal with any anxiety you may experience during a test?
   a. jogging
   b. listening to music
   c. practicing deep breathing and imagery
   d. asking for more time to take the test

Key Terms

Match the following terms with their correct definitions.

____ 1. Ability

____ 2. Anxiety

____ 3. Attitude

____ 4. Attribute

____ 5. Encoding

____ 6. Learning

____ 7. Learning Disability

____ 8. Learning Style

____ 9. Metacognition

____ 10. Mnemonic

____ 11. Perfectionism

____ 12. Procrastination

____ 13. Time Management

a. System to help meet goals through problem solving.

b. Method to aid in association and recall; a memorable sentence created from the first letters of a list of items to be used to recall the items later.

c. Act or process of acquiring knowledge and/or skill in a particular subject.

d. Physiologic response of the autonomic nervous system to a perceived stressful situation.

e. Process of examining the way we think.

f. Intentionally putting off or delaying something that should be done.

g. Characteristic that belongs to an individual.

h. Heterogenous group of disorders manifested by significant difficulties in the acquisition and use of listening, speaking, reading, writing, reasoning, or mathematical abilities.

i. Overwhelming expectation of being able to get everything done.

j. Individual preference for receiving, processing, and assimilating information about a particular subject.

k. Laying down tracks in areas of the brain to enhance the ability to recall and utilize information.

l. Manner, feeling, or position toward a person or thing.

m. Competence in an activity.

Abbreviation Review

Write the meaning or definition of the following abbreviations, acronyms, and symbols.

1. BP _____

2. CAI _____

3. NCLEX-PN _____

Exercises and Activities

1. In the first diagram on the top, fill in each of the smaller boxes with skills you believe are useful or necessary to be a competent nurse. Then do the same in the second diagram by filling in skills that you will need to be a successful student.

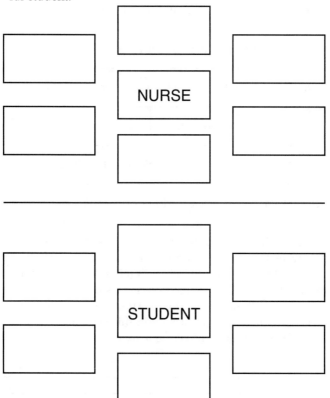

2. Using the following list of skills in the first column, write at least three examples of how each skill might be used in nursing in the second column.

Skills	Examples in Nursing
Reading	
Mathematics	
Writing	
Listening	
Speaking	

3. Rewrite each of these negative statements into positive ones that encourage problem solving and goal-oriented behavior.

    a. "I can't understand math equations."

    _____

    b. "I have too much homework to do."

    _____

    c. "I can't stay awake in that class."

    _____

    d. "I don't understand what the teacher is saying."

    _____

    e. "The teacher goes through the material too fast."

    _____

    f. "I'm never going to be able to learn all of this."

    _____

    g. "I know I'm going to do poorly on this exam."

    _____

4. Reread the descriptions of the two classroom settings in your text on page 52. Professor A uses a variety of teaching techniques, and Professor B relies on a straight lecture format. Now imagine that you are a student in Professor B's class. List several strategies that you could use to enhance your learning in this class. Include ideas that relate to different learning styles.

    _____

    _____

    _____

    _____

5. Use the following time graph and personalize it for yourself for your class and clinical schedule. Don't forget to
   include class time, lecture and clinical work, religious activities, family commitments, study time, and transportation.

   Sunday   Monday   Tuesday   Wednesday   Thursday   Friday   Saturday

   7 A.M. _____

   8 A.M. _____

   9 A.M. _____

   10 A.M. _____

   11 A.M. _____

   12 P.M. _____

   1 P.M. _____

   2 P.M. _____

   3 P.M. _____

   4 P.M. _____

   5 P.M. _____

   6 P.M. _____

   7 P.M. _____

   8 P.M. _____

   9 P.M. _____

   10 P.M. _____

   11 P.M. _____

What is your best study time?
Is that reflected in your schedule?

   List three personal time wasters for you and one strategy
   for each that could help you reclaim some of that time.

   Time Waster   **Strategy**

   (1)

   (2)

   (3)

   List two activities that you could delegate to others.

   (1)

   (2)

6. As a new LP/VN, you are caring for your client, Mrs.
   Thompson, a new mother who delivered her first baby
   yesterday evening. You note that Mrs. Thompson appears
   to be somewhat tired this morning, but very excited about
   her new baby. Although somewhat nervous about caring

for her new baby, she asks you to show her how to give a bath. The baby is awake but quiet—this is the perfect time. What teaching strategy could you include for each of the following learning styles to help Mrs. Thompson learn how to bathe her baby?

Visual: _____

_____

Auditory: _____

_____

Kinesthetic: _____

_____

Self-Assessment Questions

1. Mild anxiety may cause a student to:
   a. be more easily distracted.
   b. focus in on small or scattered details.
   c. feel alert and motivated.
   d. lose a sense of the "whole."

2. It is crucial that a student who may have a learning disability:
   a. focus on application of information.
   b. develop alternative learning styles.
   c. become a kinesthetic learner.
   d. get professional testing.

3. Being able to summarize a writer's message shows evidence of:
   a. basic competency.
   b. accuracy.
   c. comprehension.
   d. metacognition.

4. A student who has practiced testing skills for the NCLEX-PN will:
   a. attempt to identify priorities correctly.
   b. infer additional data from experiences.
   c. first scan questions to determine difficulty level.
   d. establish agreement or disagreement with the question.

5. A nurse caring for several ill patients with multiple needs may rely primarily on:

   a. skill building.
   b. time-management skills.
   c. help from colleagues.
   d. goal setting.

6. A student who is learning to give an injection demonstrates a kinesthetic learning strategy by:

   a. studying injection techniques with a small group of students.
   b. watching a nurse give an injection to a client.
   c. demonstrating an injection on a laboratory mannequin.
   d. developing a chart on various types of injection techniques.

⚡ WEB FLASH!

- Visit your professional association's web site and gather information on your profession.
- Visit one of the learning sites to take a learning-style assessment.

Critical Thinking Questions

In the section on Practicing Thinking Critically, you were asked, "How did you arrive at that conclusion?" Recall the last fairly crucial decision you made and outline your thinking process.

References/Suggested Readings

Alfaro-Lefevre, R. (1999). *Critical thinking in nursing: A practical approach* (2nd ed.) Philadelphia: W. B. Saunders Company.

The Center for New Discoveries in Learning, Personal Learning Style Inventory/School Smart Kids. (1998). *Newsletter*, Vol. 1. No. 4 [On-line]. Available: http://www.howtolearn.com/ndil3.html

Chaffee, J. (1999). *The thinkers guide to college success*. Boston: Houghton Mifflin Company.

Chopra, D. (1997, May–June). How can I keep up? *Natural Health,* 208.

Dale, E. (1954). *Audiovisual methods in teaching.* New York: Dryden Press.

DeLaune S., & Ladner, P. (1998). *Fundamentals of nursing: Standards & practice.* Albany, NY: Delmar.

DeWit, S. (1999). *Saunders student nurse planner.* Philadelphia: Saunders Co.

Dirkx, J., & Prenger, S. (1997). *A guide for planning and implementing instruction for adults—A theme-based approach.* San Francisco: Jossey-Bass.

Dunn, R. (1996, January). How learning style changes over a period of time. *InterEd* [Special edition], 3–4.

Harrington, N., Smith N., Spratt W., & Walker, L. (1996). *LPN to RN transitions.* Philadelphia: Lippincott-Raven.

Hoffman, K. (1997). *Effective college planning* (5th ed.). Orchard Park, NY: WNY Collegiate Consortium of Disability Advocates.

Holkeboer, R., & Walker, L. (1999). *Right from the start.* Belmont, CA: Wadsworth Publishing Company.

Knowles, M. (1988). *The modern practice of adult education. From pedagogy to andragogy.* Englewood, NJ: Cambridge.

Korchek, N., & Sides, M. (1998). *Successful test-taking: Learning strategies for nurses* (3rd ed.). Philadelphia: Lippincott Williams & Wilkins.

Lagerquist, S., & Billings, O. (1996). *Little, Brown's nursing Q&A critical thinking exercises.* Boston: Little, Brown and Company.

Lesar, I. S. (1998). Errors in the use of medication dosage equations. *Archives of Pediatric Adolescent Medicine, 152*(4), 340–344.

Matthews, K. H. (1997, Fall). Learning out of the box. Tuning in to your unique cluster of intelligences. *The Next Step Magazine,* 22–27.

Meltzer M., & Palau, S. M. (1996). *Acquiring critical thinking skills.* Philadelphia: Saunders.

Meltzer M., & Marcus-Palau, S. (1997). *Learning strategies in nursing. Reading, studying and test taking* (2nd ed.). Philadelphia: Saunders.

Meltzer M., & Palau, S. M. (1998). *Learning strategies for allied health students.* Philadelphia: Saunders.

Mind tools: How your learning style affects your use of mnemonics. (1998). [On-line]. Available: http://www.mindtools.com/mnemlsty.html

National Center for Learning Disabilities (NCLD) Inc. (1999, January 24). *Information about learning disabilities* [On-line]. Available: www.ncld.org

Nugent, P., & Vitale, B. (2000). *Test success: Test taking techniques for beginning nursing student* (3rd ed.). Philadelphia: F. A. Davis.

Rubenfeld, M. G., & Scheffer, B. (1998). *Critical thinking in nursing: An interactive approach* (3rd ed.). Philadelphia: J.B. Lippincott Williams & Wilkins.

Schank, R. (2000). *Dynamic memory revisited* (2nd ed.). Cambridge, UK: Cambridge University Press.

Scott, A., & Fong, E. (1998). *Body structures and functions* (9th ed.). Albany, NY: Delmar.

Smith, G. L., Davis, P. E., & Dennerll, J. T. (1999). *Medical terminology: A programmed systems approach* (8th ed.). Albany, NY: Delmar.

Sotiriou. P., & Phillips, A. (1999). *Steps to reading proficiency* (5th ed.). Belmont: Wadsworth Publishing.

Resources

Agency for Healthcare Quality and Research, www.ahqr.gov

The Institute for Learning Sciences, 1890 Maple Avenue, Evanston, IL 60201, 847-491-3500, www.ils.nwu.edu

Identifying Your Best Learning Styles, http://marin.cc.ca.us/~don/Study/13styles.html

Mind Tools: The Old School House, Yapton, West Sussez, United Kingdom, BN18 ODU

Mind Tools: How Your Learning Style Affects Your Use of Mnemonics. www.mindtools.com/mnemlsty.html

The Center for New Discoveries in Learning, P.O. Box 1019, Windsor, CA 95492, 707-837-8180

The Center for New Discoveries in Learning Personal Learning Style Inventory/School Smart Kids Newsletter Vol. 1, No. 4, www.howtolearn.com/ndil3.html

National Center for Learning Disabilities, Inc., 381 Park Avenue South, Suite 1401, New York, NY 10016, 212-545-7510, 888-575-7373, www.ncld.org/

The National Adult Literacy and Learning Disabilities Center (National ALLD), Academy for Educational Development, 1875 Connecticut Avenue, NW, Washington, DC 20009-1202, 202-884-8185, 800/953-ALLD (953-2553), FAX: 202/884-8429, http://novel.nifl.gov/nalldtop.htm

Choosing a College for Students with Learning Disabilities. www.ldresources.com/collegechoice.html

Directory of Adaptive Technology: Trace Research and Development Center, 5-151 Waisman Center, 1500 Highland Avenue, University of Wisconsin, Madison, WI, 53705, 608-262-6966, http://trace.wisc.edu/CRERO/trace.html

Closing the Gap, A Resource Directory, P.O. Box 68, 526 Main Street, Henderson, MN 56044, 507-248-3294

Appendix A: Nursing Practice Standards for the Licensed Practical/ Vocational Nurse

Nursing Practice Standards is one of the ways that NFLPN meets the objective of its bylaws to address principles and ethics and also to meet another Article II objective. "To interpret the standards of practical (vocational) nursing."

In recent years, LPNs and LVNs have practiced in a changing environment. As LPNs and LVNs practice in expanding roles in the health care system, *Nursing Practice Standards* is essential reading for LPNs, LVNs, PN, and VN students and their educators, and all who practice with LPNs and LVNs.

NURSING PRACTICE STANDARDS FOR THE LICENSED PRACTICAL/ VOCATIONAL NURSE

Preface

The Standards were developed and adopted by NFLPN to provide a basic model whereby the quality of health service and nursing service and nursing care given by LP/VNs may be measured and evaluated.

These nursing practice standards are applicable in any practice setting. The degree to which individual standards are applied will vary according to the individual needs of the patient, the type of health care agency or services and the community resources.

The scope of licensed practical nursing has extended into specialized nursing services. Therefore, specialized fields of nursing are included in this document.

THE CODE FOR LICENSED PRACTICAL/VOCATIONAL NURSES

The Code, adopted by NFLPN in 1961 and revised in 1979, provides a motivation for establishing, maintaining, and elevating professional standards. Each LP/VN, upon entering the profession, inherits the responsibility to adhere to the standards of ethical practice and conduct as set forth in this Code.

1. Know the scope of maximum utilization of the LP/VN as specified by the nursing practice act and function within this scope.
2. Safeguard the confidential information acquired from any source about the patient.
3. Provide health care to all patients regardless of race, creed, cultural background, disease, or lifestyle.
4. Refuse to give endorsement to the sale and promotion of commercial products or services.
5. Uphold the highest standards in personal appearance, language, dress, and demeanor.
6. Stay informed about issues affecting the practice of nursing and delivery of health care and, where appropriate, participate in government and policy decisions.
7. Accept the responsibility for safe nursing by keeping oneself mentally and physically fit and educationally prepared to practice.
8. Accept responsibility for membership in NFLPN and participate in its efforts to maintain the established standards of nursing practice and employment policies which lead to quality patient care.

Introductory Statement

Definition

Practical/Vocational nursing means the performance for compensation of authorized acts of nursing which utilize specialized knowledge and skills and which meet the health needs of people in a variety of settings under the direction of qualified health professionals.

Scope

Practical/Vocational nursing comprises the common core of nursing and, therefore, is a valid entry into the nursing profession.

Opportunities exist for practicing in a milieu where different professions unite their particular skills in a team effort for one common objective—to preserve or improve an individual patient's functioning.

Opportunities also exist for upward mobility within the profession through academic education and for lateral expansion of knowledge and expertise through both academic and continuing education.

Standards

Education

The Licensed Practical/Vocational Nurse

1. Shall complete a formal education program in practical nursing approved by the appropriate nursing authority in a state.
2. Shall successfully pass the National Council Licensure Examination for Practical Nurses.
3. Shall participate in initial orientation within the employing institution.

Legal/Ethical Status

The Licensed Practical/Vocational Nurse

1. Shall hold a current license to practice nursing as an LP/VN in accordance with the law of the state wherein employed.
2. Shall know the scope of nursing practice authorized by the Nursing Practice Act in the state wherein employed.
3. Shall have a personal commitment to fulfill the legal responsibilities inherent in good nursing practice.
4. Shall take responsible actions in situations wherein there is unprofessional conduct by a peer or other health care provider.
5. Shall recognize and have a commitment to meet the ethical and moral obligations of the practice of nursing.
6. Shall not accept or perform professional responsibilities which the individual knows (s)he is not competent to perform.

Practice

The Licensed Practical/Vocational Nurse

1. Shall accept assigned responsibilities as an accountable member of the health care team.
2. Shall function within the limits of educational preparation and experience as related to the assigned duties.

3. Shall function with other members of the health care team in promoting and maintaining health, preventing disease and disability, caring for and rehabilitating individuals who are experiencing an altered health state, and contributing to the ultimate quality of life until death.

4. Shall know and utilize the nursing process in planning, implementing, and evaluating health services and nursing care for the individual patient or group.

   a. Planning: The planning of nursing includes:
      1) assessment of health status of the individual patient, the family and community groups
      2) an analysis of the information gained from assessment
      3) the identification of health goals.

   b. Implementation: The plan for nursing care is put into practice to achieve the stated goals and includes:
      1) observing, recording and reporting significant changes which require intervention or different goals
      2) applying nursing knowledge and skills to promote and maintain health to prevent disease and disability and to optimize functional capabilities of an individual patient
      3) assisting the patient and family with activities of daily living and encouraging self-care as appropriate
      4) carrying out therapeutic regimens and protocols prescribed by an RN, physician, or other persons authorized by state law.

   c. Evaluations: The plan for nursing care and its implementations are evaluated to measure the progress toward the stated goals and will include appropriate person and/or groups to determine:
      1) the relevancy of current goals in relation to the progress of the individual patient
      2) the involvement of the recipients of care in the evaluation process
      3) the quality of the nursing action in the implementation of the plan
      4) a re-ordering of priorities or new goal setting in the care plan.

5. Shall participate in peer review and other evaluation processes.

6. Shall participate in the development of policies concerning the health and nursing needs of society and in the roles and functions of the LP/VN.

Continuing Education

The Licensed Practical/Vocational Nurse

1. Shall be responsible for maintaining the highest possible level of professional competence at all times.
2. Shall periodically reassess career goals and select continuing education activities which will help to achieve these goals.
3. Shall take advantage of continuing education opportunities which will lead to personal growth and professional development
4. Shall seek and participate in continuing education activities which are approved for credit by appropriate organizations, such as the NFLPN.

Specialized Nursing Practice

The Licensed Practical/Vocational Nurse

1. Shall have had at least one year's experience in nursing at the staff level.
2. Shall present personal qualifications that are indicative of potential abilities for practice in the chosen specialized nursing area.
3. Shall present evidence of completion of a program or course that is approved by an appropriate agency to provide the knowledge and skills necessary for effective nursing services in the specialized field.
4. Shall meet all of the standards of practice as set forth in this document.

GLOSSARY

Authorized (acts of Nursing) Those nursing activities made legal through State Nurse Practice Acts or other laws.

Lateral Expansion of Knowledge An extension of the basic core of information learned in the school of practical nursing.

Peer Review A formal evaluation of performance on the job by other LP/VNs.

Specialized Nursing Practice A restricted field of nursing in which a person is particularly skilled and has specific knowledge.

Therapeutic Regimens Regulated plans designed to bring about effective treatment of disease.

Upward Mobility A change of career goal, e.g., Licensed Practical/Vocational Nurse to Registered Nurse.

LP/VN A combined abbreviation for Licensed Practical Nurse and Licensed Vocational Nurse. The LVN is title used in California and Texas for the nurses who are called LPNs in other states.

Milieu One's environment and surroundings.

Protocols Courses of treatment which include specific steps to be performed in a stated order.

Would you like to know more about the National Federation of Licensed Practical Nurses, Inc.?
For information about NFLPN and how you can become a member, write to NFLPN at the address shown below:

NFLPN
893 US Highway 70 West, Suite 202, Garner, N.C. 27529

or contact us by telephone:
(919) 779-0046 • (800) 948-2511 • Fax (919) 779-5642
www.nflpn.org

Appendix B: Answer Key

Note: Answers to the Exercises and Activities are individualized to each student

CHAPTER 1 CRITICAL THINKING

Review Questions

1. A branch of learning or field of study is called a:
   d. discipline.
2. Fundamental to quality thinking is the ability to think:
   a. clearly.
3. The person who is concrete or exact when stating or applying a fact is practicing the standard for critical thinking called:
   d. specificity.
4. The person who has the ability to separate needed information from information not needed at the present time is practicing the standard for critical thinking called:
   b. relevance.
5. Ideas or things that are taken for granted are called:
   c. assumptions.
6. The person who is willing to take an unpopular position based on reasoning is said to have:
   a. courage.

Key Terms

1. f	7. h
2. c	8. k
3. d	9. b
4. g	10. i
5. j	11. e
6. a	

Abbreviation Review

1. Universal Intellectual Standards

Self-Assessment Questions

1. a	5. c
2. c	6. d
3. d	7. b
4. a	

CHAPTER 2 SKILLS FOR SUCCESS

Review Questions

1. Ninety percent of your program is based on which basic skill?
   c. reading
2. What is the sign of true comprehension of material?
   d. the ability to summarize the material using your own words
3. If you suspect you have a learning disability, it is important that you:
   b. be tested to determine the assistance you will need to compensate for the disability.
4. A kinesthetic learner:
   b. learns by movement and imitation.
5. The best way to study is to:
   c. read, reread, reflect, recite, and review.
6. What is the best way to deal with any anxiety you may experience during the test?
   c. practicing deep breathing and imagery

Key Terms

1. m	8. j
2. d	9. e
3. l	10. b
4. g	11. i
5. k	12. f
6. c	13. a
7. h	

Abbreviation Review

1. blood pressure
2. computer-assisted instruction
3. National Council Licensure Examination—Practical Nursing

Self-Assessment Questions

1. c	4. a
2. d	5. b
3. c	6. c

Glossary

Ability Competence in an activity.

Anxiety Subjective response that occurs when a person experiences a real or perceived threat to well-being; a diverse feeling of dread or apprehension.

Attitude Manner, feeling, or position toward a person or thing.

Attribute Characteristic that belongs to an individual.

Concept Mental picture of abstract phenomena that serves to organize observations related to those phenomena.

Critical Thinking Mode of thinking—about any subject, content, or problem—whereby the thinker improves the quality of his or her thinking by skillfully taking charge of the structures inherent in thinking and imposing intellectual standards (or a level of degree of quality) upon them.

Discipline Branch of learning, field of study, or occupation requiring specialized knowledge.

Disciplined Trained by instruction and exercise.

Encoding Laying down tracks in areas of the brain to enhance the ability to recall and utilize information.

Judgment Ability to evaluate alternatives to arrive at an appropriate course of action.

Justify To prove or show to be valid.

Learning Act or process of acquiring knowledge and/or skill in a particular subject.

Learning Disability Heterogenous group of disorders manifested by significant difficulties in the acquisition and use of listening, speaking, reading, writing, reasoning, or mathematical abilities.

Learning Style Individual preference for receiving, processing, and assimilating information about a particular subject.

Logic Formal principles of a branch of knowledge (such as nursing).

Metacognition Process of examining the way we think.

Mnemonic Method to aid in association and recall; a memorable sentence created from the first letters of a list of items to be used to recall the items later.

Opinion Subjective belief.

Perfectionism Overwhelming expectation of being able to get everything done.

Procrastination Intentionally putting off or delaying something that should be done.

Reasoning Use of the elements of thought to solve a problem or settle a question.

Reflective Introspective.

Standard Level or degree of quality.

Time Management System to help meet goals through problem solving.

Index

Note: Page numbers in **bold type** reference non-text material.

30-second vacation, anxiety and, **80**

A

Abilities, recognizing, 39–41
Accuracy vs. inaccuracy in thinking, 13
Adequacy vs. inadequacy in thinking, 15–16
Anxiety
  30-second vacation and, **80**
  reducing, 79–81
Arithmetic, as a basic skill, 46–47
Assumptions, reasoning and, 18
Attitude
  basic skills development and, 43–52
  competency list, **44**
  chart, **38**
  defined, 37
  developing a positive, 37–52
  positive self-image and, 37–39
  realistic expectations and, 41–43
  recognizing abilities and, 39–41
Attribute, defined, 37–39
Auditory learners, **55**

B

Basic skills
  arithmetic/mathematics and, 46–47
  competency list of, **44**
  comprehension, strategies to improve, **46**
  development of, 43–52
  listening as, 47–50
  reading as a, 44–46
  speaking as a, 50–52
  writing as, 47
Bias vs. fairness in thinking, 16

C

Calendar, week-at-a-glance, **60**
Center for Critical Thinking, 4

Clarity vs. lack of clarity in thinking, 11–12
Clutter, as a time waster, **60**
Commitments, analyzing, 59, 61–62
Completeness vs. incompleteness in thinking, 15
Comprehension
  importance of, 45
  strategies to improve, **46**
Concept, of critical thinking, 2
Concepts, reasoning and, 20
Conclusions, reasoning and, 20–21
Consequences, reasoning and, 21
Consistency vs. inconsistency in thinking, 14
Courage, disciplined thinker and, 22
Critical listening, 9
Critical reading, 6–8
Critical speaking, 10–11
Critical thinking
  activity and, 5–6
  defined, 1, 4
  described, **21**
  discussed, 2–6
  new information and, 5
  nursing and, 23
  practicing, 76–77
  skills of, 6–11
    listening, 9
    reading, 6–8
    speaking, 10–11
    writing, 10
  standards for, 11–16
    accuracy vs. inaccuracy, 13
    adequacy vs. inadequacy, 15–16
    clarity vs. lack of clarity, 11–12
    completeness vs. incompleteness, 15
    consistency vs. inconsistency, 14
    depth vs. superficiality, 14–15

fairness vs. bias, 16
logical vs. illogical, 14
precision vs. imprecision, 12
relevance vs. irrelevance,
  13–14
significance vs. triviality, 15
specificity vs. vagueness, 12
student responsibility for, 6
Critical writing, 10

D

Data, reasoning and, 19–20
Depth vs. superficiality in
  thinking, 14–15
Discipline, defined, 2
Disciplined, defined, 2
Disciplined thinker, traits of,
  21–23

E

Essay test strategies, 87–88
Exams, preparing for, 74–75
Expectations, identifying realistic,
  41–43

F

Fairness vs. bias in thinking, 16

G

Goals, clarifying, 62–63

H

Heaslip, Penny, 4
Humility, disciplined thinker
  and, 22

I

Illogical vs. logical thinking, 13–14
Implications, reasoning and, 21
Imprecision vs. precision in
  thinking, 12
Inaccuracy vs. accuracy in
  thinking, 13
Inadequacy vs. adequacy in
  thinking, 15–16
Incompleteness vs. completeness
  in thinking, 15
Inconsistency vs. consistency in
  thinking, 14
Inferences, reasoning and, 20–21
Information
  critical thinking and, 5

reasoning and, 19–20
Integrity, disciplined thinker
  and, 22
Intellectual standards, defined, 2
Interruptions
  minimizing, 67
  as a time waster, **60–61**
Introspection/reflection in
  thinking, 2
Introspective thinking, 2
Irrelevancy vs. relevance in
  thinking, 13–14

J

Judgments, defined, 6
Justify, defined, 14

K

Kinesthetic learners, **55**

L

Learners, types of, **55**
Learning attitude, appropriate,
  64–65
Learning, defined, 35
Learning disabilities, **53**
Learning environment, setting
  up, 65
Learning, strategies for, 56–57
Learning styles
  classification of, 54–56
  developing positive, 52–54
  division of, **55**
  strategies and, **58**
Lectures, attending, **75**
Listening
  as a basic skill, 47–51
  critical, 9
Logical vs. illogical thinking, 14

M

Matching test strategies, 87
Mathematics, as a basic skill,
  46–47
Metacognition, 76
Mnemonics, **72**
Multiple-choice test strategies,
  87

N

NCLEX-PN, 75
Note taking, 71–74

Nursing, critical thinking in, 23
Nursing process, critical thinking and, 23
Nursing standards/practice guidelines, 23

O

Opinions, defined, 6

P

Perfectionism, 42
  behaviors of, **43**
  as a time waster, **61**
Perseverance, disciplined thinker and, 22–23
Point of view, reasoning and, 19
Precision vs. imprecision in thinking, 12
Priorities, setting, 63–64
Problem-solving, reasoning and, 16–21
Procrastination, as a time waster, **61**
Purpose, reasoning and, 18

Q

Quality thinking, 4
Question at issue, reasoning and, 18

R

Reading
  as a basic skill, 44–46
  critical, 6–8
  strategic list of, **7**
Reason, disciplined thinker and, 22
Reasoning
  assumptions and, 18
  concepts and, 20
  data/information and, 19–20
  defined, 4
  elements of thought in, **17**
  implications/consequences and, 21
  inferences/conclusions and, 20–21
  point of view and, 19
  problem-solving and, 16–21
  purpose of, 18
  question at issue and, 18
Reflective thinking, 2

Relevance vs. irrelevance in thinking, 13–14
Resources, gathering, 66–67

S

Self, knowing, 62
Self-discipline, time-management and, 64
Self-image, developing a positive, 37–39
Short answer test strategies, 87
Significant vs. triviality in thinking, 15
Skills
  arithmetic/mathematics as a basic, 46–47
  development of basic, 43–52
    competency list, **44**
  listening as a basic, 47–50
  reading as a, 44–46
  reading as a basic, 44–46
  speaking as a basic, 50–52
  test-taking, 78–88
  writing as a basic, 47
Speaking
  as a basic skill, 50–52
  critical, 10–11
Specificity vs. vagueness in thinking, 12
Standards
  intellectual, 2
  nursing, 23
Study, appropriate learning attitude, 64–65
Study plan, setting up, 68–71
Superficiality vs. depth in thinking, 14–15

T

Test Question Analysis Worksheet, **82**
Testing room, behaviors in, 85–86
Test-taking skills
  additional data, do not infer, 84
  anxiety reduction and, 79–81
  attitude/expectations and, 78
  improving, 81–85
  know the material, 85
  preparation and, 78–79
  priorities, identify correctly, 84–85

read carefully, 83–84
strategies and, 86–88
Test Question Analysis
  Worksheet, **82**
testing room, behaviors in,
  85–86
vocabulary and, 84
Textbooks, becoming familiar
  with, 67–68
Thinker, traits of a disciplined,
  21–23
Thinking
  assessing our own, **3**
  critical, 2–6
    accuracy vs. inaccuracy, 13
    activity and, 5–6
    adequacy vs. inadequacy,
      15–16
    clarity vs. lack of clarity,
      11–12
    completeness vs. incom-
      pleteness, 15
    consistency vs. inconsistency,
      14
    depth vs. superficiality,
      14–15
    fairness vs. bias, 16
    logical vs. illogical, 13–14
    new information and, 5
    nursing and, 23
    practicing, 76–77
    precision vs. imprecision, 12
    relevance vs. irrelevance,
      13–14
    significance vs. triviality, 15
    skills of, 6–11
    specificity vs. vagueness, 12
    standards for, 11–16
    student responsibility for, 6
  quality, 4
  reflective/introspective, 2

Time commitments, analyzing,
  59, 61–62
Time wasters, **60–61**
Time-management, 57–64
  appropriate learning attitude
    and, 64–65
  commitments and, 59, 61–62
  defined, 57
  gathering resources and,
    66–67
  goal clarification and, 62–63
  knowing self and, 62
  lecture attendance and, **75**
  minimizing interruptions and,
    67
  mnemonics and, **72**
  note taking and, 71–74
  preparing for exams and,
    74–75
  self-discipline and, 64
  setting priorities and, 63–64
  study environment and, 65
  study plan and, 68–71
  textbooks and, 67–68
  time wasters and, **60**
Triviality vs. significant in
  thinking, 15
True/false test strategies, 87

V

Vagueness vs. specificity in
  thinking, 12
Visual learners, **55**
Vocabulary, importance of, 45

W

Week-at-a-glance calendar, **60**
Writing
  as a basic skill, 47
  critical, 10
  steps to clear, **49**